THE

SOFTBALL

TRIP

A story of players learning to become
better teammates and leaders.

Jamy Bechler & Michael K. Thompson

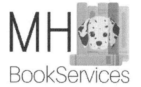

Chapter discussion guides are available at
JamyBechler.com/Resources

The Softball Trip is a work of fiction designed to help individuals
understand how to be better teammates and more positive leaders.
This book is based upon and adapted from *The Bus Trip* by Jamy
Bechler. Names, characters, businesses, organizations, places, events,
incidents, or locales are the product of the author's imagination or are
used fictitiously. Any resemblance to actual persons, living or dead, or
locales is entirely coincidental or intended to honor those people and
inspire people to make the world a better place.

FROM JAMY ...

Thanks to my wife Tabitha for your love, support, and encouragement. This book would not have been possible without you. I love you.

Thank you to Jaylen for being the greatest son a dad could ask for.

FROM MICHAEL ...

Thank you to my parents, Curt and Louise Thompson. They've supported me through thousands of games as a player and coach. In every kind of Michigan weather, my parents are there to support me unconditionally.

I'm thankful to my brother Brian and sister Kelly for their support & encouragement in writing this book. A special thank you to my brother Gerry, who demonstrated courage & bravery in his battle with brain cancer. I look forward to the day we can play another football game in Heaven's front yard.

I also want to express my deep gratitude to the thousands of players I have been fortunate to work with, past and present. You have not only taught me about the game but also about life. The game is not just about winning or losing but about the relationships we build. We have shared countless moments of joy and sorrow, and I am grateful for each one. The memories we created on our Florida trips, bus trips, and on the field will always hold a special place in my heart, just as you do.

I have also enjoyed working with some of the finest coaches and teachers. Thank you for your dedication to working with students, and I am grateful for your friendships and camaraderie.

A special thank you to my 11th-grade English classes for their patience and honesty in their feedback. Their input about food, the language, coffee, and 21st-century pop culture made this book easier to complete.

A huge thank you to my co-author, Jamy Bechler, for the amazing opportunity to write this book with him and for the chance to share some of my stories. I am excited to see how The Softball Trip will inspire and impact the next generation of players and teams.

Lastly, I want to honor my good friend Darrin Batdorff, who the coach in this book is named after. Darrin was a fantastic person and fellow coach who fought the brave fight against cancer. Thank you for the memories and your commitment to education and athletes.

This book is dedicated to all the athletes striving to be great teammates and leaders. Leaders make people and situations better, so regardless of your role, status, talent, or age, you can be a person of influence. Stay encouraged and keep doing what's right. Integrity is not situational.

CONTENTS

WAKE UP

*J*ust *a small town girl / Living in a lonely world / She took the midnight train going anywhere.*

"Seriously, shut that thing off!" shouted Kylee.

The alarm was too loud and went off too early in the morning. But Piper knew it was the exact time it needed to go off because it was the very time she set it for.

"Are you deaf? Shut that thing off!"

Kylee meant business and wasn't a fan of Piper's alarm clock, regardless of what she set the ringtone to.

Piper hit the off button.

"Yeah, it was a little loud. But regardless, we need to get up. Game Day, right?!?" Piper said as she threw off her blanket and hopped out of bed.

"That's what they say. But it doesn't matter for some of us, remember? Some of us have the best ticket in the ballpark. The far end of the dugout!"

"Whatever, Captain."

"Captain of the dugout steps, you mean."

Even though Kylee had been a highly recruited athlete, she had failed to live up to her potential through the years. She was now barely playing even though she was a captain. Her position was due

1

more to her status as one of only two seniors on the team rather than anything she had done to be a good team leader.

On the other hand, even though Piper was not a captain, she had earned the respect and admiration of seemingly everyone. She had invested the time to get to know each of her teammates and knew what made each of them tick. Piper knew the birthday and middle name of every single player.

"I just know that we've got to get up now because we didn't give ourselves much time to mess around before we needed to be on the bus," said Piper.

"Maybe, but it's not like it'd be the worst thing in the world to get left behind. Then I could enjoy a day off and not have to put up with another loss and the embarrassment of not playing again."

Piper glared at Kylee with disapproval and disdain. As the team's lead-off hitter and starting center-fielder, the junior took every loss personally.

"Let's focus on what we need to do today," Piper said gently.

"What we need," said Kylee. "Is a break from this season."

"We'll all get a break soon enough," said Piper, shaking her head at her roommate. "But we've still got a month before the season is over, and until then, we need to get dressed and head over to the field. Like it or not, we do have another game today. It might be the same old, same old for some, but this is what we do. I, for one, can think of hundreds of worse things to do than playing softball and hanging out with friends all day."

With that, Kylee and Piper got dressed and left the dorm. It had seemed as if they had gone through this routine a million times, but little did they know that this day would not be like all the rest.

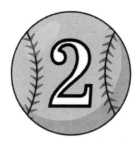

LOADING UP THE BUS

For more than a decade, Ben Batdorff had counted the Eagles when he got on the bus. He loved leaving early if possible, but he also wanted to make sure that he didn't leave players behind if they left early.

"I counted," proclaimed Coach Batdorff. "Who are we missing?"

"You're joking, right coach?" asked Andrea. "We're missing the usuals."

By the usuals, Andrea meant Gretchen and Libby. Those two had a habit of being late for everything. They seemed to operate in a world devoid of time, clocks, or calendars.

"Well, they still have a couple of minutes," said Coach Batdorff.

"One of these days, they are going to cut it too close and totally miss the bus," said Andrea.

"We'll deal with that when it happens. For right now, we're lucky that it hasn't happened yet."

"Even though they're our starting pitcher and catcher, we've been losing, so maybe it wouldn't be so bad if they finally cut it too close," said Andrea. "Maybe our luck would change."

"Our problems are not because of two players," responded Coach Batdorff. "Our struggles this year have gone a little deeper than that."

Gretchen and Libby were similar players on a softball diamond in terms of their athleticism and versatility. They were both returning all-conference players. Libby was Gretchen's pitcher. That's the way she viewed her role. Pitchers belonged to her. Unfortunately, their pitching/catching combination wasn't the only thing they had in common. In addition to being late more often than not, they tended to think the world revolved around them both.

Though Coach Batdorff was facing the back of the bus, talking with Andrea and some other players, he knew precisely the moment that Gretchen and Libby boarded the bus.

"Let's go and crush it!" Gretchen announced loudly.

"Lessgo! Let's get this show on the road," said Libby, as the two seemed to feed off one another.

There was certainly no questioning their enthusiasm. Even amidst a losing streak, they were boisterous and energetic. Many of their teammates silently questioned their motives for being so enthusiastic.

"Good morning, ladies," said Mr. Frank.

"Good morning, Mr. Frank," the players said in unison.

Mr. Frank had been driving the team for years. He had seen Coach Batdorff and the Eagles experience a lot of success. Unfortunately, this season had been the most challenging Mr. Frank had observed throughout the years of serving as the Eagles' bus driver.

"You ready to be the best you can be today?" asked Mr. Frank.

"You know it! Ready to throw darts," said Libby.

"I hope so," Mr. Frank responded. "Your team needs your leadership today."

"Don't worry about that. We're ready to get after it. They can't stop us. We're getting a win today," Gretchen boasted confidently.

"Glad to hear that, ladies. But you know I'm not talking about you throwing strikes. Just throwing strikes doesn't make you a leader, and trying to hit home runs every at-bat isn't always what your team needs, but I'm sure you'll figure it out. Today is a bright, beautiful day. Great day for us to count our blessings."

"Mr. Frank, you say that to us every time we get on this bus. Instead of calling you Mr. Frank, we should call you Mr. Rainbows and Butterflies. You're one positive guy," said Libby.

"I try to be, ladies. There's just too much negativity in this world. I want to see you girls be the best you can be. Now, speaking about being the best you can be, you had better hustle to your seats. Now, as you said when you got on the bus a few minutes ago, 'It's time to get this show on the road.' But, then again, you already know it's time to go because when you get on the bus, it's always time to go. Literally."

"Wait, did I detect a little sarcasm there, Mr. Frank?" asked Libby.

With a smile and in his own little awwhh shucks sort of way, Mr. Frank said, "You caught me. My wife says I'm doing better with that, but I still need to watch myself. Now get on the back to your seats. This bus is itching to hit the road."

Coach Batdorff moved to the side as Gretchen and Libby walked past, barely acknowledging him.

"Well?" asked Coach Batdorff.

"Well, what?" responded Libby.

"We've been waiting on you ladies. Is your time more valuable than ours?"

"We had to grab our coffee, and there was a line at the shop. You want us to be well caffeinated, right, Coach?" asked Gretchen.

"I don't mind your coffee and want you to play well. But, they have coffee at the dorm."

"Yeah, but they don't make the iced mocha I like," Libby pointed out.

Gretchen spoke up. "And the dorm's attempt at a caramel frappe is an embarrassment to the university."

"Iced mocha and caramel frappe?" asked Coach Batdorff.

Libby and Gretchen just stared at Coach Batdorff. They didn't really care what he had to say about this issue and were hoping that the question he just asked was rhetorical. They also wished he would soon be done talking so they could continue to their seats.

Coach Batdorff tried to make his point. "Maybe if you give yourselves extra time getting your precious juice, you wouldn't put all the consequences of your lateness on us."

"Maybe, Coach, but why don't you just get the university to expand its coffee offerings? Win-win, right?" replied Libby.

Coach Batdorff tended to be more patient than some other coaches, but that was put to the test often when dealing with Libby and Gretchen.

"A real win-win would be you ladies arriving when your teammates get here, and then everybody can leave on time, and you don't have to get lectured by me. Win-win-win! Now, please go sit down. We're already running a couple of minutes late. We have to get moving."

With that, the two players continued past Coach Batdorff, rolling their eyes and joining their teammates as Mr. Frank navigated the bus out of the parking lot.

ARRIVAL

This was the kind of trip that Mr. Frank liked. It was all freeway, and there was very little traffic this morning. They would soon be arriving at their destination.

"We're 30 minutes from the field," Coach Batdorff announced. "Everyone, wake up, get out your scouting reports, and let's go over them one last time before we get to the stadium. Make sure to note, again, their pitching tendencies, spray charts, and bunt coverages. This team we're playing doesn't cover the bunt well. I really think we can take advantage of them with small ball."

Most of the players reached into their backpacks for their scouting reports and started mindlessly reading through them.

"You know what one of the best things about not playing much is?" Ava asked her roommate, Zoe. "Scouting reports don't matter to me. I don't have to stop watching TikTok on my phone when Coach says to go over scouting reports."

"What if something happens and Coach has to put you in?" joked Zoe. "Won't you need to know what's going on?"

"That's funny. If I get into the game, it's over, and it won't matter who's pitching, who's in the outfield, at the corner spots, or even behind the plate. Especially how weak they are in defending the bunt. When I get into the game, it's never when the game is on the line. I just hit bombs or balls to the gap. That's my role. Don't ask me to do anything else. Coach doesn't give me many chances or whatever you want to call it. For me, it's 'don't matter time' for Ava."

Zoe just looked at her roommate with a mix of sadness and astonishment and said, "Just trying to help. I want to see you ready in case your opportunity comes."

"My opportunity came when I was being recruited, and I didn't choose someplace else. That's what I should've done. Coach isn't giving me any chances here. But I'm stuck now. Between my major and the fact that I haven't put up any stats, I can't leave now."

"I wouldn't want you to leave. I'd have to find a new roommate. Think of how scary that would be, especially if my new roommate didn't have a car. How would I possibly get to Walmart?"

Zoe and Ava chuckled at that thought. Zoe began looking at her scouting report, and Ava clicked on the next TikTok video of funny cats she was watching.

The two players had clicked on Zoe's visit last year. They played the same position and were both exceptional outfielders. Even though they were competing for the same job, they ended up bonding over things outside of playing time and minutes. Even though Ava wished she were playing more, she didn't seem to be jealous of Zoe or hold it against her in any way.

Nearly thirty minutes later, Coach Batdorff announced that they'd arrived. He gave the team final instructions about getting to the locker room, where the training room was, and when they'd need to be ready for pre-game warmups.

"Remember, just because we've lost a few games lately, this is a game that we can win. It's a good matchup for us. We've given you everything you need to know in those scouting reports. Prepare yourself mentally. In the next seven innings, we will break this losing streak. Now, let's go."

After half-listening to Coach Batdorff's instructions, the players exited the bus, sure they knew the outcome already.

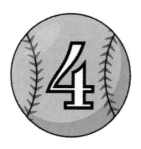

POST-GAME

It was a scene that had repeated itself far too often this season for the Eagles. The players filed into the visitor's locker room, took their seats, and waited for Coach Batdorff to explain why they lost another game to another team with less talent.

"I know we've lost games this year, but that might have been the most disappointing loss yet," Coach Batdorff lamented. "We couldn't throw strikes. We didn't make routine plays. We swung at pitches outside the strike zone and watched the ones down the middle. The dugout had zero energy. Not a single one of your uniforms is dirty. We just didn't care. They played badly, yet we weren't ready to capitalize on that. That was our chance to get a win, and instead, we went ahead and did nothing. I can't believe what I saw out there."

He pursed his lips and pondered what to say next to his group of dejected players.

"I truly don't know what to say anymore," continued Coach Batdorff. "We're not going to practice tomorrow. As players, you need to regroup, and we coaches need to meet and decide what we're going to do now. I don't normally like to cancel practice because it will only give us one practice before our next game. I don't even know if you care about that game, even though it's against our rivals. But regardless, there will be no practice tomorrow. Hopefully, you come back ready to get after it in our one practice before taking on the Lakers."

He thought he saw some players slightly smile at the thought of not having practice.

Coach Batdorff said, "The bus will roll out in 45 minutes. Get a quick shower, get dressed, get ice on your arms, and do whatever you need to do, but don't lollygag. I don't want to be here any longer than we need to. Remember to pick up all your trash in the locker room. Now, bring it in."

"1, 2, 3, Team," and with one of the weaker-sounding huddle breaks one will ever hear, a frustrated Coach Batdorff walked out of the locker room and slammed the door.

"No practice tomorrow is just fine with me," said Andrea as she hurriedly dressed and left the locker room with a massive smile.

"She might be fine with no practice tomorrow, but I guess getting three hits like she did makes her feel better," said Gretchen as some of her teammates nodded in agreement. "None of the rest of us did much of anything at the plate. We had a chance at a big inning, but..." Gretchen cut herself off.

Over in the corner, Libby sat with her head in her hands after her poor pitching performance. When she looked up, she looked at her hands, wondering if they had oil on them. Not only did she have terrible control over her pitches, but she also struck out three times.

"Keep your head up," said Haley, one of the co-captains. "You'll do better next time. It was just one bad game. None of us played well. I had a ball hit to me at shortstop that I misplayed. I own that mistake."

"Pfft. You can't win league MVP if you walk that many kids and don't produce at the plate! I'm grateful Coach lets me hit as a pitcher. Most pitchers don't. But, think what today did to my batting average," said Libby.

"I imagine it's also pretty hard to be the Most Valuable Player if you're on a losing team," Haley pointed out.

Gretchen stood up. "We all played badly even with Andrea's three hits. Quit feeling sorry for yourself. You still probably lead the league in batting average. A few more games like that, though, and I might catch you."

Gretchen continued, "Shoot, now that I think about it, Andrea might even catch up to you."

"I know you guys don't like making errors and not getting hits, but remember, that's not the ultimate goal," Haley reminded them. "Sure, we all want to hit home runs and improve our averages, but winning should be important, not your stats."

Haley put her batting helmet into her bag and addressed the girls one last time.

"Now, as Coach said, let's clean this place up, get on the bus, and get out of here."

PARENT CONFRONTATION

Coach Batdorff exited the locker room with the box score in his hands. Though the numbers told an ugly story about today's game, he knew the answers to the team's season-long woes were not contained in that paper.

"Coach, you got a minute?" It was Kylee's dad, Greg, and he didn't look happy.

"Not really," said Coach Batdorff. "Can we set up a time to talk tomorrow afternoon? Let me know what time is good, and I can call you."

"No, we need to talk now! You're not treating my daughter very well. You've shown me time and time again that you don't care about her, and you refuse to give her opportunities even though she is a captain. That actually makes things worse. How can you sit your captain?"

"I appreciate your concern for Kylee. I know she appreciates your support of her and her teammates by attending all these games, but there is a better time and place to discuss this. I'd be glad to..."

Coach Batdorff wasn't able to finish as Kylee's dad interrupted him.

"No, this is exactly the time and place. My daughter doesn't need to get lost any deeper in your doghouse. You need to understand how your coaching is affecting her."

It was evident to Coach Batdorff that Kylee's dad was getting increasingly heated, and he needed to defuse the situation.

"We don't have practice tomorrow, so that'd be a great time to talk. We'll both be less emotional, and we can talk through some things. Let me ask you, what's the thing you're most frustrated with right now, and we'll be sure to address that tomorrow?"

"That's easy. Kylee is a senior leader. She told me that you called for her to hit for Jasmine with the bases loaded. Then you went with someone else instead. That was embarrassing!"

"For you or Kylee?" asked Coach Batdorff.

"It doesn't matter. You just don't treat people that way."

"Well, I'll be glad to talk with you tomorrow about your perception of how I treat Kylee. As you point out, we'll also need to discuss her questionable attitude and lack of engagement despite being a captain. But specifically, regarding tonight, I actually called for Kylee twice. From my spot as the third base coach, I called her number 7 and tapped on my head. That is my signal that number 7, your daughter, needs to get her helmet on and get ready to hit. She was looking down and apparently didn't hear or see me. So, I called, again, 'Seven' louder and tapped my head. Again, she seemed to be engaged with something and didn't see or hear me. So, I called 'Nine' and went with another hitter."

"Well, she tells me you were too far away for her to hear."

"Did your daughter tell you what she was actually doing when I tried to put her in the game, Greg, and 'didn't hear me?' My manager told me that Kylee was looking up concert tickets that had just gone on sale today."

"It seems to me that you were disrespectful to her. How do you take out a senior for a freshman?"

"Disrespectful, do you say? Did Kylee ever tell you that being on your phone and not engaged in the game was one of my non-negotiable behaviors? Did she ever tell you that that type of behavior could get her dismissed from the team?"

Just then, Mr. Frank approached the two men.

"Sorry to interrupt, fellas, but Coach, the trainer needs to talk about Piper's leg with you. I'm sorry about that. I'm sure you fellas can catch up tomorrow or the next day."

"Thanks, Mr. Frank," said Coach Batdorff.

As he turned to head toward the training room, Coach Batdorff said, "Greg, please text me and let me know when you want to talk tomorrow."

Once Coach Batdorff had walked away, Mr. Frank turned his attention to Kylee's dad.

"Hey, Greg. Good to see you. I hope that I didn't interrupt anything too pressing."

"Well, I've been frustrated all year, and it came to a head tonight. It's probably good that you came when you did," said Kylee's dad.

"Why's that, Greg?" Mr. Frank asked him.

"I might have jumped to conclusions too quickly or at least been wrong on one thing. I'm not super happy, but I need some time to think about what Coach said."

"Well, glad to hear it. I know we've been friends for a while, and you love Kylee, but I also know that you want the team to succeed. Part of that is at least giving Coach a chance to explain things and discuss things with you. I hope you fellas can work it out tomorrow. Like I said, good to see you, and have a good trip home."

"You too, Frank. Don't drink too many of those energy drinks. You'll have to make way too many pit stops," Greg said with a wink.

TRAINING ROOM

Although Coach Batdorff was glad to be leaving the situation with Kylee's dad, he dreaded what awaited him as he headed toward the athletic training room.

"How's Piper?" Coach Batdorff asked Angela.

Angela had been the Eagles' trainer for many years. She was very good at what she did. Angela was knowledgeable and extremely caring. She had a great mix of personality and wisdom. She could put players and coaches at ease but also knew where the boundaries were. She was a true professional, and the Eagles were lucky to have her.

"It's not good," Angela replied. "We won't know for certain until tomorrow when we can get an MRI, but I'm guessing that it's completely torn, and she'll miss the remainder of the season."

Coach Batdorff's heart dropped. The season had been challenging enough, even with Piper as the leadoff hitter and centerfielder and doing all she could to help the team. She always did what Coach asked, and she did it with a smile. She wasn't the most gifted, but she was intelligent, rugged, and had a positive attitude. It seemed like everyone liked Piper. It still amazed him that Piper and Kylee were roommates. They were polar opposites with their attitudes and sense of responsibility.

"I'm really sorry about this, Piper. Hang in there," said Coach Batdorff.

"I just can't believe my season might be over. This hasn't been a good year, but I was determined to do all I could to help us on the field to finish strong," said Piper.

"I know that. Let's wait and see what the doctor says tomorrow," said Coach Batdorff. "But, if it's torn and you're out for the rest of the season, you can still help us turn this season around. We only have about six weeks left, but we have enough games to finish strong. You might not be able to lead on the field, but you can certainly lead from the dugout."

"Thanks, Coach. I will do what I can."

"I know you will. You control the controllable, Piper, and you definitely know how to bring energy and positivity to the team. You can do that wherever you are, whether on the field, the classroom, or the dugout."

Angela brought over some crutches and handed them to Piper.

"I think Piper can serve as a good role model for the team," she said. "And you're right. She'll provide enthusiasm and energy even though she isn't playing. I think she can be infectious but in a good way."

Coach Batdorff nodded in agreement and patted Piper on the back, "I'll see you on the bus."

After Coach Batdorff had left the training room to go to the media center, Angela, Piper, and Tracy were the only Eagles remaining in the training room.

"I can't believe you got hurt," Tracy said from another training table. "You bring so much energy to the team. You've got to be the hardest worker I've ever been around. Your effort is incredible. Day in and day out, it doesn't matter."

"I appreciate that, Tracy. But I don't do anything special. I've always played hard because I knew that my softball career would be over one day, and I didn't want to look back and have any regrets.

Looks like my season might be over a little sooner than expected, but I still have no regrets other than I wasn't able to help us get more wins."

"You did what you could," said Tracy. "But maybe the season isn't over. Maybe you'll just be out for like a week or something."

"Hope so, but the reality is that Angela is pretty good at what she does, and she has prepared me for the possibility that I'm done. She thinks that even if it isn't officially torn all the way, it might be difficult to return from this in the month or so we have left in the season. I'm mentally preparing myself so that this is probably it for me."

Piper was tough and had a good attitude, but it was evident that the thought of missing the remainder of the season was difficult for her. She was trying to stay optimistic around Tracy. She knew Tracy looked up to her ever since Piper hosted Tracy on a recruiting visit last year. Tracy came from a good background. She was a solid player and a good student. Piper could see a little bit of herself in Tracy as she didn't excel at anything and didn't have many obvious flaws.

"You're the energy for our team. I'm not sure what we'll do without you. It certainly won't be the same," said Tracy.

"But, it can be. What I bring to the team is probably the easiest skill a person can have. Giving consistent effort and providing energy is something that anyone can do regardless of size, athletic ability, status on the team, or batting average," Piper pointed out.

"You say that, but if it's so easy, why don't more players bust their tail like you do?" Tracy asked.

"That's a great question," said Piper. "Unfortunately, I was never as naturally gifted in hitting or fielding as Gretchen or pitching like Libby. I had to find other ways to make myself valuable. Certainly, I knew a positive attitude could help, but I had to do more. I had to go further than that. I had to find a way to turn that positive attitude into a softball skill. I figured that I could outwork other people. That's how I landed a job as a leadoff hitter and centerfielder."

Piper adjusted the ice pack on her knee before continuing her answer.

"I figured I could hustle on the field. I could be aggressive on the bases. If I practiced diving for balls, tracking balls in the outfield, and building my arm strength to throw to bases, I would have an advantage over others. I could make up for my average speed if I became a better baserunner. Speed kills, it's true, but some girls with speed are horrible baserunners. They don't anticipate very well."

"I wish that I could do what you do."

Piper responded to Tracy, "That's the thing. What I do shouldn't be special. Anyone can do it. You definitely can do it. It's a mentality. It's me saying every day that I will compete on every pitch, every at-bat, every inning. It's me saying I will get every fly ball and steal the next base in front of me. It's me saying that I will fire up our team through my play on the field."

Though Tracy hadn't thought of all this in the way Piper was explaining it, she was locked in on what she was saying. It sounded so simple as she listened to Piper break it down.

"I always think in terms of what can I do today that will bring us momentum?" continued Piper. "You can do that very thing, too. It's baby steps. You build habits, practice after practice, and play after play. It starts with deciding that you want to be someone who puts forth effort and brings energy. It's all a choice."

"But, I don't really play much," Tracy stated.

"How we perform in games is usually a direct reflection of how we've prepared," Piper responded. "You build habits daily, not in just a day. You can decide today that you'll be this way, but you must recommit to that mentality and go out and do it each day. Being early for class, doing all your coursework, having a sensible social life, and staying connected with your family. Those things apply to our sport. Be early for practice and stay late. Ask for extra reps. Seek out help from experienced players. Have coaches hit you extra balls and throw you extra pitches. Work on being a well-rounded person and a well-rounded player. It starts in practice, and the things we do every day, at six in the morning and midnight, will eventually become automatic for you. Your success is a choice."

"I definitely could improve in those areas," said Tracy.

"We all can do better," admitted Piper. "It's hard to be a spectator from the dugout and watch hitters have lousy at-bats. But when we have a mentality that every pitch is a strike until it isn't, it's easier to react. Some players struggle when overthinking at the plate or get distracted playing in the field. Failure is part of the game. Our choice in how we react is what matters."

"Wait, what? How is that possible? I've got to hear this one."

"Well, think about it," Piper said. "Softball is a game of failure. Let me give you an example. My grandfather was a big fan of a baseball player named Ted Williams. Ted was an amazing hitter. On the last day of the season in 1941, Ted could have sat out and preserved his .400 batting average. Instead, he chose to play both games of the doubleheader, went 6 for 8, and finished the season with a .406 batting average. No major league baseball player has ever finished a season with a .400 batting average since Ted Williams."

"Wow," said Tracy. "He took a big risk."

"Sure, he did. But that's not my point." Piper paused. "Even the best hitters, like Ted Williams, fail more than they succeed. A .406 average batting means he got a hit about 40% of the time. That also means that the guy with the best single-season batting average in the history of Major League Baseball failed about 60% of the time."

"I never really thought of that stuff," said Tracy.

"The truth is that .406 batting average is Ted's 'outcome.' It's the 'process' that is important. Have quality at-bats. Swing at good pitches. Hit to all fields. Work off the tee. Take an extra bucket at batting practice. Those are things that you can control. If you do those things, you'll see your average increase. Coach will have more confidence in you, call for you more often, and you'll feel better about yourself because you're contributing to the team's success. It's really just a mindset."

Tracy shook her head. "You make it sound so easy."

"Even the best hitter will be off some days. There will be some days when the ball just doesn't bounce our way. Balls we drive hard find their way into someone's mitt, or players make great plays. But my hustle and effort will never have an off day. I determine my effort. Not the coach, not the umpires, not my teammates, and not the circumstances. I'm the only one that can control how hard I work," Piper pointed out.

"Even though I'm a freshman riding the bench, I think I can start doing some of the stuff you said. I'm going to try it," said Tracy.

"When I was a freshman, I experienced some of the same things that you may struggle with," said Piper. "It was a big jump up in level of play, and some of the things I did in high school didn't work as easily at this level. I wasn't playing as much as maybe I expected coming out of high school. Let me tell you what Coach did my freshman year that I'll never forget."

SPARK PLUG

A ngela came over and replaced Piper's ice pack with an elastic wrap and a knee brace that would temporarily secure her knee until they returned to their home training room. Piper thanked her and then continued telling Tracy about her freshman year.

"Anyway, Coach knew that my dad was into cars, so he took a shot that I knew something about cars. He asked me what my dream car was. I told him that it was a Lamborghini. He told me something that I'll never forget. He told me a little spark plug costing five to ten dollars could keep that rich man's car from running. On the flip side, that little inexpensive spark plug can deliver electric current from the ignition system to the combustion chamber."

"You kind of lost me there at the end. Sorry, I'm not much of a car girl. I don't know a battery from a carburetor," Tracy asked, obviously confused.

"Sorry about that," apologized Piper. "A spark plug is just something that provides a spark. It ignites an engine. It provides energy. Even an expensive car can't run without it. Our team might be talented, but if not for the energy, if not for spark plugs, then individual talents on a team are wasted. Without a spark plug, a Lamborghini sits useless in the garage. Every car needs spark plugs. Every team needs them, too."

"So, you're the spark plug on this team?" asked Tracy.

"Well, I'm one of them," Piper replied. "The best teams have lots of spark plugs. The best teams have everyone giving energy and effort. I do what I can as a leadoff hitter. Hitting is contagious. I know my teammates have a better chance if I get on base first. I hope my play inspires and motivates others to play harder, but I can't make you or anyone else want it. You've got to decide for yourself. I do hope, though, that my style of play and effort can be infectious, in a good way, like Angela said earlier."

Angela was packing up some equipment in the corner but was still listening to the conversation. She smiled when she heard her mention what she'd said earlier. It always made her feel good when the players listened to what she said. She cared about the student-athletes. Not only did she want them to be physically strong and healthy, but she wanted them to develop as people.

Piper continued, "We're either energy givers or takers. We can be a vampire and suck the life out of the team or be an oxygen mask, breathing life into the team. We can complain, go through the motions, do the bare minimum, or we can make others better. We can be positive. We can try to generate momentum even when things seem at a standstill. No matter our talent, we can always provide energy."

"I've seen your success with working so hard," said Tracy. "It's got to be worth it."

"This could very well be your time," Piper replied. "With me out, we will need a new leadoff hitter: someone savvy, courageous, and willing to be the sparkplug."

"You really think I can be that person?" Tracy replied doubtfully.

"Just look at some of the best players in the world," said Piper. "They aren't lazy. They don't take plays off. There are plenty of talented players that don't fulfill their potential. Everyone in college is talented. Everyone in the NFL, NBA, or any other professional league like Athletes Unlimited are talented. What separates the best? What takes certain players from good to great? Talent is never enough. If you combine talent with effort and energy, now you've got the potential for a great player."

Angela finished putting the last piece of equipment into the sports medicine travel bag and approached the two players.

"I have the luxury of watching everything from a distance and observing," noted Angela. "Piper certainly works hard. Her energy can be contagious. Some other players occasionally do this, but they aren't consistent. Piper brings it every day, not just when she's feeling good. A few times, she's been sick or not feeling good, and you wouldn't have known it. Tracy, if you want this mentality Piper talks about, you can do it. It's your choice. It might not get you into the lineup immediately, but it'll be another step closer to getting this team where it needs to be."

"What do you mean?" asked Tracy.

"Have you ever been to a huge professional sporting event where they do the wave?" asked Angela.

Tracy nodded her head up and down. Growing up, she'd been to many Saturday afternoon tailgates and college football games with her dad and brothers.

Angela continued, thinking, "I bet you've never seen an announcement on the big jumbotron asking you to do the wave. You've probably never heard the announcer tell you it was time for the wave."

"Now that you mention it, I haven't. How do those things start?" Tracy asked.

"Great question. That's my point," said Angela. "It starts with one or two people getting one or two people to do it with them. Then another couple of people start to do it, and then more. Eventually, you have a whole section and another, and the whole stadium is doing the wave."

"All because one drunk yahoo started the wave?" asked Tracy.

"Right, except they don't necessarily have to be drunk, or a yahoo, for that matter," replied Angela. "If you want to influence your team, whether you're playing or not, and you want to be a valuable part of this team, then, be that person that starts the wave. Be the person that ignites and energizes your team. Be the cheerleader on the top step of the dugout. Be the change that you want to see on this team."

Piper said, "Be a yahoo, Tracy! Start the wave on our team."

"There's that, but in listening to you talk, Tracy, not just today, but at other times, I believe you want more for this team," continued Angela. "If that's the case, let that change start with you. It might be more important than ever now that Piper is hurt. Somebody has to pick up the baton and run with it. Somebody has to be the player that takes over as the spark plug on the field. If not in games, at least in practice, where you can build positive habits. Who knows, maybe you'll get the other yahoos in the other stadium sections to follow your lead."

"I think I can be the yahoo this team needs," Tracy said with a smile.

"Awesome," said Piper. "I guess I have a new partner in crime when trying to infect our teammates with enthusiasm, energy, and a desire to work hard."

"I'm in. Thanks for talking to me, Piper," said Tracy. "Also, thank you, Angela, for inspiring me to be a yahoo."

"You're welcome," said Angela. "Now, you two better get out of here and on that bus. You don't want Gretchen and Libby to get on first."

LEAVING THE FIELD

When Coach Batdorff got on the bus, it was noisy. Players were interacting loudly, music was being played that should have been quieted by headphones, and there were plenty of cell phone conversations that should have stayed private.

It was bad enough that they just lost a game in an embarrassing fashion, but then he was unfairly confronted by a parent. To top it all off, Piper was most likely out for the season. Now he had to put up with Katy Perry on the bus.

It wasn't even an hour since his locker room tirade. He had no choice but to wonder if they even cared at all.

"Quiet down back there!" demanded Coach. "At least act like you care that we lost tonight."

"We care," responded Zoe, genuinely.

Zoe, I want to believe you, he told her silently. You're a freshman and have the right mentality. I have high hopes for you. You have a bright future. Please don't let the bad habits of some of our team "leaders" affect your potential.

"You might care, but it's obvious that most of your teammates don't care," Coach Batdorff said to Zoe.

He then turned his attention to everybody again.

"Y'all think you care. But if you truly did, then you'd act like it. We just lost a game we shouldn't have lost, and nobody would know it by how you're behaving right now. Most people might even think you won. You don't care. You're not focused. You're not committed. I'm not even saying that just because of how you're acting right now on the bus. It's more than that."

Frustrated and flushed, overwhelmed by his emotions, Coach Batdorff had not been able to figure out this team as he had done with past teams. Everything came to a head, and he had to get a few more things off his chest that he hadn't said in his short post-game locker room talk.

"If you actually cared, you'd stand up for people when they come to the dugout after leaving the field. You'd help teammates get their mitts, and their bats, and encourage them. You'd practice hard so that you could play hard. You'd act like champions instead of just participants. Sometimes, I think this is just glorified travel ball. I don't see any commitment because none of you have invested anything. I see only selfishness."

The bus was silent except for the sound of the diesel engine.

The scorebook Coach Batdorff was looking at after the game told him about outcomes. It was clear the reasons behind many of those numbers and results were often because of the very things he was talking about now.

Coach Batdorff continued, "You ladies say you care, but you just glance over scouting reports. You don't get enough sleep at night. You criticize one another. You criticize coaches. You don't pull for each other during batting practice. When someone makes a mistake, everyone has an excuse: 'The umpire made a bad call.' 'My boyfriend and I had a fight.' 'Coach is picking on me.' You don't take practice seriously. You don't run the bases hard. You don't 'wear your effort' by diving for balls. All the motivation comes from the coaches, not yourselves. Sure, you do what is asked of you, but nothing more. You hold back your energy because you don't want it badly enough."

Even though he had everyone's attention now, he decided to use a slightly different approach as he continued.

"Have any of you ever heard of the Spanish explorer Cortez?" he asked.

Silence.

"Way back in the day, Cortez and his men landed in Mexico and were attempting to colonize that land for Spain, but they had to face the mighty Aztec Indians. He sensed that his men were a little bit fearful. To motivate them, Cortex ordered that all the boats be burned. There was no turning around. No turning back. Retreat was not an option. They were all-in. They had each other's backs because there wasn't an alternative. That's a real commitment."

Coach Batdorff might have been finished with the Cortez story, but he wasn't done trying to make his point. There was still enough time left in the season for a turnaround. He didn't know if this particular team could change their mentality, but he was determined to keep trying to inspire them.

Coach Batdorff continued, "How many of you fully bought in? How many of you are willing to go the extra mile for your teammates at practice and in class? How many of you don't need someone looking over your shoulder 24/7 to make sure you did your workout? How many of you look at what you do every single day as an investment in yourself and your team? How many of your hearts are really in it? How many of you hold each other accountable?"

More silence.

Does what I'm saying make any sense to them? Coach Batdorff thought silently. Am I just wasting my breath? I care about this team, these ladies, and their success. But, I have to remember that they are young.

"Most people don't outwork their talent, ladies. The best players in the world are the best, not because they are talented, but because they maximize their talent by outworking their talent. Even if you can hit the ball to the moon, or throw the ball through the wall, you can always work harder than your baseline talent. By outworking your talent, average players can become good, and good players can become great."

I have their attention, Coach thought. Say what you have to say.

"What about us?" Coach Batdorff asked the team as they all sat in their seats. "So far this year, all you've done is the bare minimum. You're just getting by. Some of you probably can't wait for the season to end. How do you think that attitude affects your play? You can't have a negative mindset and, at the same time, be positive in your lives. Do you know what the best do better than everyone else? They come early, stay late, and do a little bit extra. They keep fighting when they're down. They refuse to quit, even if things don't go their way. They don't see obstacles, distractions, or impossibilities because they're too focused on their goals. What they want most is much more important than what is easiest right now. They know their priorities and are committed to them!"

What was once a noisy bus just minutes earlier was now eerily quiet. The players sat silently in their seats. Some of them digesting what Coach Batdorff had just said, while still a few just waited anxiously for him to finish so they could go back to their own cares and concerns.

"Coach, can I say something?" asked Mr. Frank.

MR. FRANK

Coach Batdorff had just said many good things, but Mr. Frank had something to share, and Coach Batdorff never missed an opportunity to let Mr. Frank speak and share some insights. He often asked Mr. Frank to say a few words. He and Mr. Frank had developed quite a feel for one another through the years. Mr. Frank always seemed to have perfect timing as he shared just the proper insight.

Coach Batdorff trusted Mr. Frank implicitly. Before becoming a bus driver, Mr. Frank had been a policeman, firefighter, and truck driver with over a million miles driven without a speeding ticket or a fender bender. He had even served humbly in local politics for many years. Even though he was getting up there in years, Mr. Frank still volunteered with Little League baseball and was involved in many civic organizations. His life had been all about making good decisions and helping others. Mr. Frank was full of wisdom, and Coach Batdorff never questioned his intentions or agenda.

"Sure, Mr. Frank. I'm betting that half of these ladies have stopped listening to what I was saying. Maybe they'll listen to you."

"Oh, I don't know about that, Coach. These ladies know you're only saying what you're saying because you care about them. You want them to be their best. But as you were talking, I thought of a story I read years ago that stuck with me and might stick with them, also."

Coach Batdorff sat down, nodding at Mr. Frank to continue.

"Ladies, I know the season hasn't gone as you wanted. Some of you might be frustrated with each other, with Coach, or with any number of people or things. I understand being frustrated. But, have any of you ever heard of Gustavo Nicolich?"

Mr. Frank could see a collective shaking of the head back and forth.

"I didn't think so. Gustavo Nicolich was a rugby player from Uragauy. In August of 1972, he was riding in a plane with his teammates to a match in Chile. The plane crashed into the snow-capped Andes Mountains above 11,000 feet. Half the original 45 passengers survived the crash. For ten weeks, they suffered intense starvation, altitude sickness, and severe weather, waiting to be rescued."

"Ten weeks?" Zoe asked. "It took that long to find them?"

Mr. Frank continued. "Well, Zoe, they would have never found them, and the rest would have died if it wasn't for Gustavo Nicolich."

"Why? What did he do?" asked Zoe.

"One of the guys on the plane had a portable radio that had survived the crash. The boys could listen to the news and keep track of the search. After eight days up on the mountain, Gustavo heard on the radio that the search had become no longer hopeful and had been called off. They stopped looking for the plane and its survivors."

"That would be a mental disaster to hear that, Mr. Frank," Zoe commented.

Mr. Frank continued. "Gustavo did the only thing he could do. He rounded up the boys and said, 'Boys, I have GREAT news. They have called off the search for us.'"

"Woah, woah, woah!" exclaimed Zoe. "That is the worst news in the world. How could he tell them it was GREAT news?"

"Gustavo told them, 'This is great news because we're going to get out of here on our own.' The courage of this one boy prevented a flood of total despair. They were focused and motivated. As a result, the boys prepared two of the strongest players to hike to the west, through some of the highest mountains in the world, to Chile. For the two boys, the odyssey seemed endless. They thought they would die in the mountains. But they only had one option: to keep walking and save their friends. And after more than a week of hiking to the west more than 30 miles, they finally reached the green valleys of Chile. They saved the remaining 14 boys still alive up on the mountain."

Mr. Frank paused, letting the story linger for a moment until Gretchen broke the silence with a comment that was probably on most of the players' minds.

"I get it, Mr. Frank," Gretchen replied. "Gustavo totally flipped the mentality of the situation. He turned a death sentence into an opportunity."

"You're right, Gretchen," Mr. Frank responded. "It was an unfortunate accident, for sure. But I remember that story every time I get frustrated with how things are going in my life. Whenever I think about quitting, pouting, or getting complacent, I remember those boys on the mountain. Flip the negative reality into a positive opportunity. The same applies to softball. Turn this losing streak into a GREAT opportunity to get better. Whenever you're playing a tough opponent, look at it as an opportunity to raise your game, win or lose. You never know when everything is going to click. You never know when the breaks will start coming your way. But if you quit. If you lose focus. If you lose hope. If you allow frustration to overwhelm you, you'll never be prepared or ready to cash in if and when your reward comes."

"Preach it, Mr. Frank! Say it a little louder for the people in the back," said Haley.

Raising his voice, Mr. Frank said, "IF YOU QUIT. IF YOU LOSE FOCUS. IF YOU…"

"Mr. Frank, I was messing with you," said Haley with a slight chuckle. "It's an expression. It's a way of saying you were spitting facts on us. I think everyone heard you the first time."

"Oh, okay. I need help keeping up with everything you ladies say. Regardless, enough with the talking. We need to get on the road so we can get some food in your bellies and feed the machines."

Coach Batdorff always appreciated the insights Mr. Frank provided throughout the years. Mr. Frank always seemed to know the right thing to say and when to say it. This story about the boys in the mountain was no exception. Coach Batdorff believed that Mr. Frank had just hit another home run with this story and that it might stick with a couple of players.

"Sounds good, Mr. Frank. Thanks for sharing."

Turning to the Eagles, Coach Batdorff said, "Let's think about the story Mr. Frank just told us and how it relates to our commitment to our goals and our commitment to each other. Also, ladies, please keep the music to a minimum."

Mr. Frank checked his mirrors and slowly edged out of the parking lot onto the road. The day had been tough already, and they still had quite a haul in front of them.

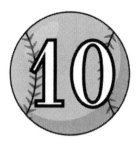

TRAFFIC JAM

It was supposed to take only 15 minutes to get from the ballpark to the Sub Shop, but as the Eagles had learned all too often this season, sometimes things could have gone better.

"We just left the ballpark, and we're already stuck in traffic. How is that even possible?" questioned Andrea.

"I know Mr. Frank is like an All-Conference bus driver, but I agree. It's weird that we're stopped already. I hope we get moving soon," Gretchen added.

The team had been consumed with other things and hadn't noticed the traffic jam for the first few minutes. Now, however, they had been stuck for ten minutes without moving an inch on this two-lane road. Ten minutes seemed like an eternity to a bunch of hungry and frustrated players.

"Why did we go this way?" Andrea continued to complain. "There had to have been a better route, right?"

"Hey, Mr. Frank, don't you have some kind of traffic app on your phone?" Gretchen asked.

"Sorry, ladies. This was the best route, but we've got a broken-down car or something like that that's pretty close in front of us. We're not on the freeway yet, so there isn't any room for us to go around. And we can't back this thing up with all the traffic behind us. We're going

33

to have to wait it out. Hopefully, it won't be much longer. Fortunately, from what I can tell, it's not a major fender-bender or anything like that. Please be patient, ladies."

"Yeah, patience is a virtue, right?" said Andrea with a hint of sarcasm.

"Yes, it is," Mr. Frank replied. "But remember that patience isn't just about our ability to wait. It's also about our attitude while we wait."

"And with that, we just got hit with another truth bomb from Mr. Frank," said Gretchen.

"Ladies, go ahead and order your subs on the Sub Shop app. That way they will be ready when we arrive. You won't have to stand in line," Coach Batdorff said. "Use your per diem."

"That's nice to be able to order in advance like that, but it doesn't put food in my stomach right now. I'm still starving," said Andrea.

"If you're that hungry, grab something from the snack box," suggested the co-captain, Haley.

"I need real food. I need more than just fruit or some crackers. I'm seriously starting to get hangry!" Andrea said irritably.

"I agree that a Spicy Italian Sub probably is better than a banana, but that's all we have right now. Guess you have a choice to make," Haley responded.

"Seriously, how does this stuff always happen to me?" moaned Andrea.

"Hey, Andrea, cut it out," Haley snapped back. "You aren't the only one that's hungry. We all are. Think of something else. Please stop talking about food; it's not helping. Mr. Frank is doing all that he can do right now. You're acting like a child. Sometimes, things that are outside our control are going to happen. Let it go."

"We could have gone a different way!" whined Andrea.

Piper had been listening to Andrea and thought of something that might help Andrea see a different perspective on their current circumstances.

"You're right, Andrea," Piper said. "But we don't know that something wouldn't have happened going that way either. Just make the best of it. Remember that sign in our locker room that says, 'Life is 10% what happens to you and 90% how you react to what happens to you'? The traffic is 10%, and your complaining is 90%."

"Hey, Andrea. Do you remember last year on the spring training trip to Florida when the TV screens weren't working?" asked Haley. "We had our student manager convinced she had to change her money into Florida money. She was so confused!"

"Yes, that was funny, not funny, because we couldn't watch TV-but still, funny," said Andrea as she remembered that bus ride.

"We made everything into a Florida-money joke for the next couple of weeks," said Haley. "Coach, did you get your Florida bills changed back to regular bills? Coach, what President is on the Florida twenty-dollar bill? Coach, will my Florida quarters work in the vending machine?" said Haley, enjoying the funny memories.

"Yeah, that was probably pretty annoying for Coach. Come to think of it, it was very mean to our manager, but I certainly got a kick out of it," said Piper.

Haley recalled, "We laugh about it now and even laughed about it then because we weren't focused on the 10%. You know, the TV was not working."

"Instead, we focused on the jokes we could make up," said Andrea.

"You're right," said Haley. "And that was the 90% the locker room sign talks about."

Just then, Piper interrupted them, "Hey, you feel that? I think we're moving again."

Indeed, the bus had started to ease forward ever so slightly, but it was progress. Slowly but surely, the bus approached a broken-down car on the road. It must have run over some nails or something because it had not one but two flat tires.

Fortunately, the driver was able to control the vehicle enough not to crash, but he couldn't get it off to the side of the road.

"Look, that car has a couple of flat tires," observed Haley.

"I'm glad we don't have flat tires," said Andrea. "We'd have waited in traffic longer, and I'd be even hungrier. Maybe now we can go get a Spicy Italian Sub."

"Sounds delicious. But I can't wait to get a veggie sub. And, do you know what, Andrea?" Haley asked.

"What?" said Andrea.

"I'm thinking that your attitude back there was similar to that car," said Haley.

"What do you mean by that?" asked Andrea.

"Well, that car couldn't go anywhere with flat tires, and you weren't getting anywhere with your bad attitude. Your attitude was like a flat tire. You can't go very far until you change it," said Haley with a smile.

"Ha, Ha. Very funny. When's your Netflix comedy special, by the way?" Andrea snapped back with a smile of his own.

"I thought it was kind of witty, but I was going for something similar to what Mr. Frank might say."

"It was close. Good try," said Andrea.

TIME TO EAT

The energy among the players was very high as they knew it was almost time to eat. Mr. Frank pulled into the restaurant's parking lot.

"Finally! I'm starving," said Andrea to anyone who would listen.

"Make sure that your travel suits are on as we go in," Coach Batdorff reminded the team. "Remember that you're representing the Eagles. Handle yourself with class."

Once all of the players and coaches had piled off the bus, Mr. Frank drove it around back, out of the way of the other customers.

Coach Batdorff thought that it was always interesting to see who rushed to the front of the line. They would all get their food quickly. In fact, they often came to this restaurant, and it never ceased to amaze him how quickly they prepared the food orders. Ordering ahead with technology was a good thing.

"Hello. My order number is 11. I used your app," said Kylee.

"What drink would you like with your combo?" asked the lady at the register.

"Sweet Tea."

"You got it."

"Thank you."

"My pleasure," she said. "I'll gladly serve the next guest."

A similar conversation repeated itself over and over again until all of the players and coaches had their trays of food and had found their seats. Actually, there was one player who didn't have her food, or at least the correct food that she ordered. Andrea approached the lady at the register.

"Hey, this isn't right," announced Andrea. "You got my order wrong."

"What seems to be the problem?" she asked.

"I ordered a Spicy Italian Sub, and this isn't a spicy sub at all," Andrea complained.

"I'm sorry about that. Did you order the pepper-jack cheese or American?"

"I ordered the American, but that doesn't even matter right now because what you gave me isn't even spicy. Never mind all the pickles, tomatoes, lettuce, and whatever else."

"I understand. I'm sorry for your inconvenience. Let me retake your order and we'll get it out to you as soon as we can," she said.

"Okay," said Andrea, shaking her head as she walked away from the counter.

Just a few minutes later, tray in hand, the lady from the register walked Andrea's food over to her.

"Sorry about the delay, and the mess up," she said. "Here's a coupon for a complimentary cookie as a small token from us to you. We regret that your dining experience wasn't what you expected."

"Yeah, thanks. I'm sure you guys didn't do it on purpose," Andrea replied. "Finally, I'm starving! I absolutely love these Spicy Italian Subs!"

It tasted as good as it always did.

Just then, Ava sat down at the table next to them and began talking loud enough for everyone to hear.

"You should have heard Zoe just now in the bathroom. She was complaining that she's never had a worse sub here than what she ate tonight. It was kind of funny. She wasn't throwing up or anything. That would have stunk if she'd had a reaction. You all know that she is a mental midget when it comes to spicy food. She's a honey mustard girl, you know. Anyway, she was complaining that her sandwich didn't taste right. She was like, 'you guys played a prank on me and traded out my salami for spicy pepperoni on my sandwich when I wasn't looking. I was sweating bullets eating that thing.' I don't know what she was talking about, but it so was funny."

Andrea interrupted, "Wait. Zoe said it was too spicy?"

"Oh, yeah. You know how soft she is. Always cheese or veggie pizza because the pepperoni is too spicy," chuckled Ava.

When Zoe came out of the bathroom, all eyes were on her.

"What?" Zoe asked, confused.

"Caliente," Ava joked.

"Oh, okay. I get it. You guys are having your fun with me," said Zoe.

"No, seriously. I'm asking for real. Was your sub actually spicy?" Andrea asked again.

"My mouth was dying but I fought through it like a champ," said Zoe. "I wasn't going to quit or give up. I was going to be like those rugby players Mr. Frank was talking about earlier tonight."

"I don't think he had your taste buds and bad food in mind when he was saying not to give up," joked Ava.

"Seriously though, back to your sub," said Andrea. "I got an absolutely boring sub, and I raised a stink at the counter. I blamed them. What was your order number?"

"Let me check," said Zoe as she looked through the crumpled-up napkins and straw wrappers on her table. "Here it is. Number nine."

"Zoe, that's a six," said Ava looking over Zoe's shoulder. "Seriously, and you're the one with a 4.0 grade point average?"

"My order number was a nine," said Andrea. "You took my food. Serves you right. No wonder it tasted spicy. It was exactly that--a spicy sub. Just like Ava said, how are you a 4.0?"

"I don't know. Let's just forget about it," Zoe requested.

"Except that I gave the lady up at the counter a hard time. I thought that they messed up the order. We were the ones that had messed things up."

"Oops," said Zoe.

"Oops, is right. I kind of feel bad," said Andrea.

Gretchen was never shy about inserting herself into a conversation, so she decided this was as good a time as any.

"You could always apologize. I've been told that is what I should do when I make my mom mad."

"Oh, you've been told, have you?" Libby asked her roommate. "I'm not sure you've ever listened to that advice. If you had, you'd probably always be apologizing for something."

Walking past Libby and Gretchen as they bantered back and forth, Andrea approached the lady from the register as she was putting away the broom and closing the storage closet door.

"Yes, ma'am. How may I help you?" she asked.

"Uhmm. Yeah, ah. I think I messed up with the Spicy Italian Sub. Sorry about that," apologized Andrea.

"What do you mean?" she asked.

"One of my teammates had it all along. I just assumed that you must have screwed up. I didn't even think it'd be my fault. Sorry about that," Andrea said.

"I understand," she said. "I'm just glad we were able to get you a replacement sub quickly enough. Does your friend need the sub that she ordered or is she okay?"

"Nah, she's good. Though it was a bit too hot for her."

"Okay, well, we just want to make sure that you have a good experience here. We take pride in our food and our service."

"I guess the customer isn't always right," Andrea said.

"None of us are right all the time. We realize that, but that doesn't stop us from still trying to serve you and find a solution to the problem if we're able to," she said.

"When you waited on me the second time, did you know that I was the one that had made a mistake?" Andrea asked.

"We don't worry about who's to blame," she said. "Life can be pretty miserable if we're always pointing fingers or playing the blame game. Instead of determining who is to blame, we try to take responsibility for things. It might not have been our fault, but we can be responsible for doing what we can to make the situation better. Fix the problem, not the blame. In your case, it was easy to make another sub."

"Thanks for that, and sorry once again," Andrea said as she turned to walk away.

"It's our pleasure to serve you," she said.

Andrea turned back toward the lady as she said that.

"Can I ask you a question?" she asked.

"Sure, what is it?" she wondered.

"You keep saying words like 'serve' and 'our pleasure.' I don't hear people at other restaurants talk like that. Why do you guys say that stuff?" asked Andrea.

"Good question. Obviously, we think we have the best subs around, but more importantly, we feel like our job here is to serve. Whether we're a new employee, a cook, someone who sweeps the floors, the manager, or the owner-no matter our role or title, we want to treat our customers like friends. We want to be kind to everyone."

The lady continued to explain to Andrea what made the restaurant different from all the others.

"You see, every life has a story. Every customer is a person. We want to go the extra mile and make someone's life a little better today. If I had worried about who was right and who was wrong about your sandwich, then I wouldn't have been trying to make your day better. I would just have tried to get my way or be right. In general, we've found that the best leaders are those who serve. People tend to follow them with their hearts and buy into what they are selling."

Andrea was still listening to the lady, and she could tell that she was interested in what she was saying.

"It might be weird or different, but I hope that it makes sense," she continued. "I might have gone a little deep on you, but I get excited talking about this stuff. I don't just work here because I want to collect a paycheck. There are plenty of jobs out there for that. I truly enjoy the people I work with but also the people---the friends, if you will---that I get to interact with every day, like you and your teammates."

"That's cool. Thanks for sharing all of that. I never really thought of any of that stuff before," Andrea said.

"By the way, what kind of cookie do you want with that coupon I gave you earlier?" she asked Andrea.

"Seriously? Even though you know that I was the one that screwed up?" Andrea said with some confusion. "Here, you can have that coupon back. Use it for someone that deserves it."

"It's not about deserving or not. We gave that to you, and we expect you to use it. You're not going to refuse us the joy of being kind to you, are you?" she asked with a sly smile. "So, what kind of cookie would you like?"

Andrea smiled. "Can I have a brownie instead?"

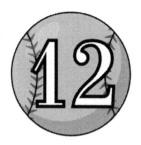

LEAVING THE RESTAURANT

As the players left the restaurant, most showed some appreciation or at least acknowledged Coach with a quick head nod as he held the door open for all of them.

"Thanks," said Andrea.

"You're welcome," said Coach.

"Don't you mean, 'My Pleasure?'" joked Andrea.

"Well played," Coach Batdorff said. "Now get on the bus. You were just almost the last one."

"Lucky for me, Gretchen and Libby are still my teammates. With them around, I'll never have to worry about being last," said Andrea as she boarded the bus.

Coach smiled as Gretchen and Libby finally strolled past him and, as usual, were the last players to board the bus.

"Hey, Coach, now that you finally decided to join us, everybody's on the bus. It's time to cook," said Gretchen as Coach got on the bus.

"Very funny," Coach snapped back.

Libby fist-pumped Gretchen and said, "We're just messing with you, Coach. We saw you walk around the restaurant, pick up that dirty napkin off the floor, and throw it away. That napkin didn't belong to any of us. That wasn't your responsibility. They hire people to do that."

"It's just the right thing to do," Coach Batdorff replied. "I don't always do what's right, unfortunately, but I still try to be a servant leader whenever possible."

"Servant leader? What does that mean? It looked like you were cleaning up after others," asked Libby.

"It really means that I'm leading by serving others," said Coach Batdorff.

"That sounds like one of those oxymorons. How can you lead and serve at the same time?" Gretchen asked.

"Serving others just means that I'm trying to help others. It means I'm trying to care for someone else's needs. Picking up a piece of trash isn't a big deal, but it's something I could do to be nice," Coach Batdorff pointed out. "In college, I worked at an amusement park during the summer. One of the things they taught us was that when we see trash on the ground, we don't think about it; we pick it up. It's just the right thing to do. When I picked up that napkin just now, it made someone else's job easier."

Andrea listened to the conversation and said, "Hey, Coach, it's funny you should say that. Do you remember when they didn't give me the right sub?"

"Yes, you seemed a little frustrated by the whole thing. But they apologized and seemed patient even though you were a little short with them," said Coach Batdorff.

"It was actually my mistake, after all," admitted Andrea. "I ended up apologizing to the checkout clerk. What's weird is that she said some of the same stuff you just said about serving and trying to improve things for others."

Coach Batdorff said, "Andrea, that lady wasn't just some checkout clerk. She's the restaurant's owner."

"Wait, what? They had a million people working there. Why was she still taking our orders and refilling our drinks? What's that all about?" Andrea asked.

"As I said, servant leadership," Coach Batdorff replied. "It's not about what she can get from the customers or her employees but how she can enrich their lives. NFL Hall of Famer Peyton Manning once said, 'The most valuable player is the one who makes the most players valuable.' When a team is more concerned about each other, they are more likely to go farther together than they could."

Coach Batdorff couldn't believe he was having this conversation with Andrea, of all people. Andrea tended to be self-focused. She might have been the most gifted softball player on the team after Gretchen and Libby, but she also knew it and, too often, acted the part of a prima donna. The fact that she was still listening and asking questions gave Coach Batdorff hope.

"Serving others doesn't mean you think less of yourself," Coach Batdorff continued. "It doesn't mean that you put yourself down. Instead, it means that you think of yourself less. You put the needs of others before your own. In turn, you improve their life, which will ultimately make your life better. You ladies share the load. You share the burdens. It's much better to go through life with friends who have each other's backs rather than worrying about your own agendas."

So far, so good, Coach thought.

Andrea looked down at her shoes in thought. Then, she looked up at Coach.

"Coach, you seem happy and proud that you picked up that garbage," Andrea said. "Why?"

Coach Batdorff replied, "There was a study done that found that we're healthier, both physically and psychologically, when we give to others and help others. It reminds me of the song from Toy Story, that says, *If you got troubles, I've got 'em too / There isn't anything I wouldn't do for you / We stick together and can see it through / Cause you've got a friend in me.*"

Libby and Gretchen gave Coach Batdorff quite the look as he recited the song lyrics, but wisely, they didn't offer an opinion on his singing voice.

"As a softball player, you can volunteer to shag balls for a teammate," he continued. "You can put balls on a tee for a teammate or throw front-toss. You can catch for a pitcher. You can hit your other infielders ground balls. You can study with a teammate. You can hold each other accountable. Keep each other out of trouble. You can do something as simple as grabbing a teammate's water bottle for them. You aren't above doing the grunt work. Find ways to help your teammates be better. This will make you better as well. No matter your age or status in life, you can always help others out. You can lean on each other."

"That's deep, Coach. I can respect that," said Andrea. "Is that why you sweep the dugout and put out all the screens before practice? I thought we had managers to do that stuff."

Coach Batdorff said, "I try to do whatever helps move our team forward, and if I can help somebody in the process, then I try to do that. As you mentioned, managers and facility employees, for example, have a lot of things to do. If I can take something off their plate, I try to do that. At the end of the day, somebody must do all these things. From a traditional way of thinking, I've certainly paid my dues and shouldn't have to do these things, but I think it's the right thing to do."

Sitting in a nearby seat, Angela, the team trainer, enjoyed this conversation. She wanted the players to be physically and mentally healthy. She felt that Andrea was learning something and was glad that Coach Batdorff was taking the time to talk with her.

When there was a slight pause in the conversation between Andrea and Coach Batdorff, Angela said, "Even though I was a biology major, I had to take some business classes. I had this one professor who gave us a test. Before giving the test, the professor said, 'I've taught you everything that I can teach you about business in the last ten weeks, but the most important message or question that I could ask would be, what's the name of the lady that cleans this building during the day? That is the only question on this test.' Even though I knew the material from the chapter, I failed that test. I think of that story often. Everybody I come in contact with is important. Everyone has a story. If I can help them in some way or treat them with kindness in some way, then I'm passing that test, so to speak. I figure that if we all help each other, then it's like iron sharpening iron. It's like Coach and the song says, 'There isn't anything I wouldn't do for you'."

Coach Batdorff added, "I know that every time you scroll through your social media feeds, it seems that you're flooded with negativity. We see people being mean. We see people being selfish. But the world is still full of people doing great things. Gandhi used to say, 'Be the change you want to see in the world.' Just because other people are negative doesn't mean we have to be. We should be kind to others, not because we get rewarded or the other person is kind, but because we're kind."

"Absolutely. Coach is right," said Angela. "Martin Luther King Jr. had a dream that people would be judged by the content of their character. The world still isn't perfect, nor will it ever be. We can't help everyone, but we can help someone. We can't do everything, but we can do something. Instead of throwing up my hands and saying that things are hopeless, I want to be the change I want to see in the world. I want to do what I can do where I'm at."

Coach Batdorff looked at Andrea and said, "Angela has great thoughts about helping others. She does that every day as our trainer. I try to be a servant leader as a coach. If that means helping others by putting out screens or even carrying bat bags, then that is what I want to do. MLK also said, *It's always the right time to do what is right.* I figure that it's always the right time to help out a custodian, manager, or anyone."

That was a lot, Coach. Do you think you and Angela have gone too far with Andrea and lost her? Coach thought.

It was quiet.

"Batdorff's deep thoughts," Andrea said, breaking the silence. "What you guys say makes a lot of sense. Now, I need to find out the name of our facility manager."

The comment eased Coach's fears. He was relieved that Andrea was responsive to their talk. Coach smiled and replied, "It's Norm, but everyone calls him Boogie."

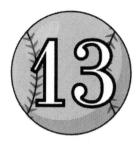

COACH'S FAVORITES

As the bus rolled along the freeway, many of the players were on their phones. Kylee was no exception. But unlike her teammates, she was the only one communicating with someone who had confronted Coach Batdorff negatively that day.

"You've been pretty quiet all night. You okay?" Haley asked Kylee, her fellow co-captain.

"Just been texting with my dad."

"I saw him and Coach talking in the parking lot after the game. Your dad looked mad. What was that all about?"

"Yeah, he got on Coach pretty hard and will be talking to him tomorrow sometime," Kylee replied. "He is going to find out why I'm not playing much. Coach has just had it out for me all year. I need a chance, but I'm not sure he will give me any."

"What was the deal tonight? I thought you were going in the game, but you didn't."

"Coach wanted me to go in, but then he chose someone else. Our manager, Kayla, was sitting right next to me, watching what I was doing. She said he called for me twice, but I didn't hear him. I ended up not playing even though the game was a blowout. I was the only one not to play. That was embarrassing."

"That stinks. Sorry. Did Coach say why he changed his mind?"

"He never said a word after the game to me. It's been like that all year. He never gives me a chance. He definitely plays favorites, and it's obvious that I'm not one of his favorites?"

"I know the season's been tough for you, but do you really think Coach plays favorites?"

"It's obvious. Of course, he does."

"I've got the solution," said Haley, as if a lightbulb had appeared above her head.

"Oh, yeah, what's that?" asked Kylee.

"Become one of his favorites. Boom! Problem solved. Next," Haley remarked with a smile.

"Not quite that simple."

"Why not?"

"Because Coach is set in his ways. It's obvious that he already has his favorites."

"Then how do you explain a couple of weeks ago when he played Jasmine, and she ended up getting that streak of hits and has yet to make an error? She's even ended up playing quite a bit since then despite being a freshman."

"Right, but Jasmine did those things. She got a chance."

"You don't remember when you had a chance around the same time?" asked Haley.

"I do. But Coach put me up against a great pitcher. He set me up to fail."

"What are you saying? You had three really bad at-bats, including taking a called third strike with the bases loaded. You just stood there and watched. Then, you almost threw the ball out of the stadium on that grounder. And, when you did hit that slow roller, it didn't look like you ran hard to first. I don't remember the last time you got extra reps in the batting cage or stayed after practice to work on your fielding. If he puts you in the game to hit off a great pitcher, he has enough faith in you that you can hit great pitching. The truth is everyone should tear up bad pitching. If you weren't ready to hit superior pitching, that is something you should work on."

"Whatever," Kylee said dismissively.

"Not whatever, Ky. Jasmine was ready for her opportunity because she worked on her game every day after practice, even though she wasn't seeing much action. She still stayed sharp. She gained confidence, but maybe, more importantly, Coach also gained confidence in her. Jasmine wasn't playing much before, but now she plays a decent amount. Even when she isn't hitting, he still has Coach's trust because Coach sees how hard she's working."

"Yeah, she's lucky to be one of Coach's favorites now."

"You're right. Jasmine's one of Coach's favorites now, but that's because she did what Coach wanted," Haley stated.

"Coach always talks about bringing energy and doing little things like diving for balls, but I think that's just talk."

"What do you mean? It seems genuine to me."

"I dove for that ball between you and me when you played shortstop a few weeks ago. That should have shown Coach that I'm serious. He talks a big game, but I didn't get rewarded. He barely acknowledged me diving for that ball. I scraped up my elbow on that one. I've also come early to practice a couple of times, but he still hasn't given me a chance," said Kylee.

"But that's not the right way to look at things. A couple of times isn't enough to earn his trust. You have to do things over and over again until he knows you're serious. It'll also start to become a habit. I saw a post on social media that I thought of when you mentioned those things. It said, 'Bad players remember the good things they do, but good players remember the times they messed up.'"

"That's one of those things that sounds good, but it doesn't matter. Coach is still going to be against me. Remember when we both missed practice, and you didn't get in trouble, but I did?"

"How could I forget? We were coming back from break for the first practice, and we were riding together. I got into trouble, but not as much as you. Remember that I had to run some sprints before I could practice?"

"We both had to run, but unlike you, I also got suspended for a game. That wasn't fair," complained Kylee.

"I don't know about that. Don't you remember when we got to the field and practice was getting over? The very first thing out of your mouth was, 'My parents didn't wake me up.' No apologies. No, nothing but blaming your parents. What are you, 12 years old? Set your own alarm clock."

"Well, I certainly didn't whine and cry for forgiveness like you did," said Kylee, mimicking a baby.

"I didn't whine quite like that," corrected Haley. "I just apologized for missing practice. I truly was sorry for that. I was also sorry that it hurt the team's preparation because someone else had to play shortstop in practice."

"You were just sorry that it made you look bad."

"Well, that might be true, also. Nobody ever wants to look bad, but that doesn't mean I was sorry."

"I've wondered something about that day. Why didn't you say it was my fault? I was your ride after all," wondered Kylee.

"True, but I chose to ride with you. I could have called you sooner when I saw you weren't at my dorm on time. But the bottom line is it didn't matter why I missed practice. I missed practice, which wasn't what I was supposed to do."

"Isn't that noble?" said Kylee sarcastically.

"Choices and actions have consequences. Sometimes good and sometimes bad. Regardless of whose fault it was, I didn't do what I was supposed to do. I was supposed to be at practice, but I didn't do that. Sure, I had a good reason for missing practice. My so-called friend was driving me and couldn't get out of bed without her parents waking her up. Talk about being a baby. But none of that matters. At the end of the day, we're responsible for controlling what we can control, and I didn't do that. There's no reason to get out of trouble or pass the buck. I just decided to own up to it and accept the consequences."

"Accept the consequences? You didn't have to do much compared to me," complained Kylee again.

"You keep saying that, and it might be true that your consequences were worse, but remember, I accepted responsibility and didn't give excuses," Haley pointed out to Kylee. "You were full of excuses and didn't accept responsibility. Besides, you had missed a couple of other practices right before break that was probably still on Coach's mind."

"Those were to take some tests. Academics first, right?" said Kylee.

"Academics first, if appropriate. I know why you were taking those tests. The professor let you make up those re-tests because you slept through the regular tests. I guess academics weren't first when it came to sleep. I also know you suggested our practice times when you could take makeup tests. That way, you could get out of practice. I heard you use that academics-first stuff on Coach when you told him you couldn't be at practice. I don't think you fooled him, but he wouldn't fight you on it."

"All of this might be true to a degree, but Coach still hasn't told me why he's not playing me more or giving me a chance in games," said Kylee.

"Don't you know what you need to do? You're not in high school anymore. You know what is right and wrong for softball players to do. Does Coach really need to spell it out for you?" asked Haley.

Kylee got defensive and responded very quickly, "He should. He should be letting me know how I can get more playing time! What does he think? Does he think I like sitting on the bench?"

"Have you asked him?" wondered Haley.

"I did back in the fall, and he just basically ignored me."

"He did? That's a little surprising."

"He said I asked the wrong question. He said he understood everybody wants more playing time, but that is a selfish question. Being consumed with playing time when you're part of a team is selfish. He said that the better question would be to ask to help me better understand my role on the team. Yeah, that pretty much ended that discussion."

"That sounds like it could have led to a longer conversation. That could have been the opening you needed to learn more about how a senior co-captain understands her role. Remember, roles are always changing. Each one of us is important. Every one of us has a role to play. If you want a role different from what you have right now, it is simple: get better," suggested Haley.

"No, it just showed me that he wasn't concerned about my playing time," Kylee snapped back.

"You're probably right about that," admitted Haley. "Coach probably doesn't care who exactly is getting playing time. He's most likely worried about the entire team. He wants the team to be as good as possible. Let me ask you a question."

"Fire away," said Kylee.

"When Coach yells at us after a game about having crappy at-bats or making too many errors, what are you thinking?" asked Haley.

"I'm wondering why he played those players that weren't getting the job done."

"What about when we get out-hustled, and he says we're being lazy?" asked Haley.

"I'm wondering why he didn't put somebody else in the game if he was so upset about the effort."

"How many games do we have in a year?"

"30-40," answered Kylee.

"How many practices, workouts, and training sessions do we have?"

"Seems like they never end. Hundreds!" exclaimed Kylee.

"Right," said Haley. "Coach is probably more likely to believe what he sees repeatedly in practice than in just one game. If the players he trusts are hitting weak grounders, pop-ups, misplaying balls in the outfield, or not putting forth the effort, he might give them a little extra leeway because he sees them doing something else in practice."

This is an important moment for Kylee, Haley thought. She is not getting upset, and she is allowing me to ask questions.

"What do you think would happen in the days following a game when Coach is mad because we played poorly, that you smoke the ball at the plate or make tons of plays in the field? What about what Coach says about 'hustle innings'? He rewards players who hustle in practice with innings in a game."

"Coach would probably notice," admitted Kylee.

"Exactly, and then you'd be on your way to being one of his favorites," said Haley. "Coach tells us all the time what being one of his favorites looks like. You don't have to guess or listen hard, even though he doesn't come right out and say it. When he mentions that the team isn't hustling, he is looking for someone to hustle. If he puts up the batting averages of everybody in the league or mentions this constantly, he values good batting averages even though we know they don't tell the whole story about our at-bats. Going to class is important if he makes a big deal of the academic honors players. Whatever he talks about the most is what he values. Give that to him. That is how you become his favorite."

"I've seen coaches act like it just doesn't matter, though," said Kylee.

"There are probably coaches like that out there, but typically, we see things only from our perspective. Remember, in high school, when I was upset with my coach because I was platooning and not batting as high up in the order as I wanted?" asked Haley.

"I do. Did you ever talk to Coach Spencer?" replied Kylee.

"I didn't. But my mom went to see him. She told him that I had more hits than so and so player, and so she couldn't understand why I wasn't getting more of an opportunity because I was clearly a better hitter. He showed her how the other kid had a way better on-base percentage, fielding percentage, and more hustle plays. Even though she was going to be out, she still ran out way more fly balls and ground outs than I did. That wasn't even something I thought the coach was paying attention to, let alone keeping stats on. He told my mom I had potential but was too focused on things I couldn't control. Instead of worrying about playing time or spot in the order, I should be hustling more, taking more fielding practice, and taking more walks instead of swinging at everything. After that conversation, I didn't complain any longer. My mom told me she would never confront a coach again, getting only one side of the story."

"Interesting story about your mom. I didn't know that. I guess talking about parents brings us back to my dad and him confronting Coach Batdorff," said Kylee. "And, I guess I should probably tell you why I didn't hear Coach call for me."

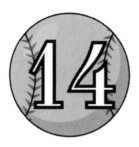

T-SHIRT

What might be unusual for some was commonplace for Haley and Kylee. Deep conversations might be avoided by many, but not them. The life-long friends had been there for each other through the good times and bad times of growing up, and they weren't afraid to tackle challenging issues along the way.

"Which brings us back to your dad," repeated Haley. "Have you been totally straight with him about your missed practices, questionable attitude, and constant excuses, AND what happened today?"

"Bruh, if you weren't my best friend...," said Kylee.

The Eagles co-captains looked at each other briefly as they considered the conversation they had been having.

"If we weren't close, I wouldn't tell you this," replied Haley. "I care about you and want you to do well. I also care about our team and want the team to do well. If you do better, then the team can do better. I also know from the situation with my mom and the high school team that we sometimes only see our side of things. Sometimes, we only see our tree and not the whole forest."

"You know you sound like Piper, right?" said Kylee as she thought about her roommate and some of the late-night conversations they had through the years. "She says some of this stuff sometimes. She doesn't bang me over the head with it like you are right now, but she gets her little digs in. Have you two been talking about me or my situation behind my back?"

"Nope, but because Piper is your roommate, she cares about you. You and I have been tight since we were kids. You know I have your back, so I must speak up. I know that you feel like you were wronged, and that you're trying to blame it on Coach, but you might be a little too consumed with that and putting your energy there instead of putting your energy toward things you can control, like your own behavior."

Haley paused momentarily, squinting her eyes and smiling as she looked at Kylee's shirt.

"I know that we think Coach is a little cheesy sometimes with his cliches or sayings. We probably haven't even given much thought to it but look at the shirts that we're all wearing. Yes, even you. You're wearing our team shirts that say 'excUses.' Have you ever thought about that? The 'u' is bigger than the other letters. What's in the middle of all the excuses? You are. We are. When we make excuses, we're the reason. We're in the middle of them. We're not taking responsibility for things. Do you remember when we traveled up north for that tournament our senior year?"

Even though it was painful at the time, Kylee now laughed at the memory.

"How could I forget that experience? It was so cold!"

"Yeah, we got upset by a team we should never have lost to," said Haley. "All we could talk about afterward was that if it hadn't been so cold, we'd have killed that team. It took me a while, but it finally dawned on me one day that they played in the same frigid temperatures. The conditions were the same for them as they were for us. We didn't play hard. We went through the motions. We made excuses. Instead of playing ball, all we could think about was getting the game over and getting warm. I remember the dugout was full of whining and excuses, and that just led us to play worse."

"I never thought of that," said Kylee.

"I love these t-shirts that coach got us. Every time I see them, I think about the excuses I've made in my life. I can't remember a single time that an excuse has gotten me closer to a goal that I had. Last summer, I saw this documentary on marathon running, and it also inspired me to eliminate excuses. Marathon runners have to run endless miles in training, most of the time by themselves, and in terrible weather. I decided that if something is important, I will find a way to get it done. If it's not important, then I will find an excuse. I think excuses are for people who don't want something bad enough."

"Alright! Seriously, enough. I get it. I'm a bad person who always has an excuse on standby," said a frustrated Kylee.

"You're not a bad person. I'm your friend and want to see you take responsibility for things you can control. You'll be much happier that way."

"Happier?!? You know how I'd be happier?" asked Kylee with a smile.

"By taking responsibility for your actions?" quipped Hayley.

"Well, there is that, but no. I thought that if I had a few more dollars in my pocket like those supermodels, that would make me happy!"

"We'd all be happier if we had more money. Way to change the subject on me."

"You noticed that huh?" said a smiling Kylee.

"Sure did. Speaking of those rich girls, though," said Haley. "Did you know that Amazon ordered something like four thousand pink iPds from Apple for Christmas a few years ago? As it turned out, Apple couldn't fulfill the order in time for Christmas. This was not good for Amazon because they had already sold all of those to their customers and were waiting for Apple to send them to Amazon. What would you have done in that situation?"

"I probably would have just apologized to my customers who were silly enough to buy a pink iPod," answered Kylee. "No one uses iPods anymore, anyway."

"That's not the point. And, yes, I'm glad we can do everything on our phones now. Apologizing to the customers might have been what I'd have done, too. It wasn't our fault that they weren't available, not because they were pink or any other color."

"Exactly. It wasn't Amazon's fault."

"You're right. It wasn't Amazon's fault, but they believed it was their responsibility to do what they could to make the situation right. What Amazon did reminds me of how we should approach softball or anything else. They took responsibility for something that happened."

"Okay, here we go," joked Kylee.

"Yes, here we go again. Just because you tried to change the subject earlier doesn't mean I'm done with you."

"Okay, I give in," said Kylee. "How did Amazon take the responsibility for Apple's mess up?"

"Amazon figured that people didn't care about why or what happened. People just want the stuff that they ordered," Haley continued. "If you advertise it, then you should have it. Amazon literally went out to stores and bought pink iPods at retail cost. They packaged these brand-new iPods in Amazon packaging and then sent them to all the customers who had preordered them."

"I bet that killed their profit margin."

"Definitely, but they figured they can make excuses or be the best, but they can't do both. True champions find ways to do what needs to be done. Amazon was willing to take a loss on an item because they were ultimately responsible for what they offered on their site. Instead of making excuses and giving lame explanations, they just found a way to get things done."

"Yes, yes, yes. I get it. Be responsible. Quit making excuses. Remember what's on the front of my team t-shirt. I get it!" exclaimed Kylee.

"And they said you were hard-headed. I don't think that's the case at all. You aren't a bad person. You'll actually listen to reason after all."

"Ha, ha, ha!" Kylee laughed mockingly, but it was evident that she was joking with her fellow co-captain.

"Since we're having a good heart-to-heart," Kylee continued. "I'm really sorry for not being engaged and looking up concert tickets on my phone during the game. They went on sale today."

"You missed out on your opportunity today," responded Haley.

"That's true," confessed Kylee. "Coach always says, 'Be ready when your opportunity comes.' I wasn't ready. I wasn't focused. Someone else got the chance, not me."

"Well, it sounds like a reasonable coaching decision, then. Coach B. was doing what was best for the team at that time."

"Truthfully, I understand it, too, Haley," Kylee replied. "It's my response which I'm not proud of."

"I was on base at the time and didn't see it," said Haley. "What did you do?"

"I slammed my helmet down and went to the end of the dugout and pouted like a child. I was angry because someone else got my at-bat, or at least what I thought should be my at bat," admitted Kylee.

"Well, that'll do it. That'll normally get a coach upset," said Haley.

"I didn't even see what Avery did when she hit for Jasmine. I said some really bad things about Coach while our manager was sitting there. I was so consumed with my feelings and my selfish emotions."

"That makes more sense now. You've got to tell your dad that. In fact, you probably need to level with him about a bunch of stuff when it comes to your playing time. Tell him you'll do better and become one of Coach's favorites. Tell him he doesn't need to talk with Coach because you haven't taken care of your business yet. You haven't controlled what you can control."

"In other words," Kylee said with a smirk. "Tell my dad I'm going to do my best to become more like Piper in how she leads and performs."

"Whatever works."

Haley looked up at the TV monitor above her seat and then back over to Kylee.

"Good talk. You know I want to help you and all. I feel that I've accomplished that mission tonight. But I've got to be honest with you. I can't be this serious much longer. It was good, and you've got a lot to think about. It would help if you controlled your behavior and reactions to things. You need to take care of yourself."

Kylee looked at her long-time friend and just shook her head. It had been a good talk, and she had a lot to think about. She didn't expect this tonight, but it could prove to be an essential conversation. Kylee's thoughts were interrupted by Haley and her parting wisdom.

"You should think about texting your dad back and telling him you'll call him at the next stop. You have a few things to discuss with him."

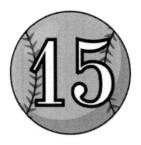

TRAVEL CENTER

M r. Frank brought the bus to a complete stop in front of the travel plaza, so it was a short walk, especially for Piper and her crutches.

"Remember to wear your travel suits and to represent our school and yourselves in a first-class manner when we go to this travel plaza," insisted Coach Batdorff. "And, remember the buddy policy. No one goes anywhere alone."

Mr. Frank added, "We'll be rolling out in 30 minutes, so please plan accordingly."

As they got off the bus, the players headed in many different directions. Some went to use the restrooms, some went to get food or snacks, but most raced to find a good place to plug their phone chargers and breathe new life into their most prized possessions.

Ava and Zoe found a great outlet right next to some very comfortable seats. They were relieved because they wouldn't have to stand for the entire thirty minutes that they were at the travel plaza.

"My mom gave me one of those power banks for Christmas, and it has been a lifesaver. I'm always prepared if I run out of juice. I always have this portable phone charger with me," said Zoe.

"I probably should get one of those, myself," Ava responded to her roommate.

"It'd be a good idea. Never be too prepared when it comes to your phone's battery. If my battery died, I don't know what I'd do. I imagine you'd be hurting if your battery were dead, or almost dead, and we didn't stop somewhere that had outlets."

"Hashtag, facts," agreed Ava.

"Speaking of being prepared," said Zoe. "Coach Batdorff might not have realized this, but in the game today, after you went in for Piper in centerfield, you were totally out of position."

"I'm pretty sure Coach noticed that."

"He probably did notice, but he probably didn't know why it happened," corrected Zoe. "What I meant was that each of those times I remember, it was something from our scouting report. If you had studied their hitting tendencies in your scouting report, you would have had the ball hit right to you and not have to try and run it down at all. That #3 hitter is a dead-pull hitter, and you should've known that. I'm guessing Coach just assumed you knew the scouting report. But I know differently. I know you didn't pay attention to that stuff or go over it. It came back to bite us. Those would have been outs if you had been in the right spot in the outfield. Instead, they were hits."

"Well, I didn't expect Piper to get hurt. I wasn't expecting to be called into action," confessed Ava.

"Those hits weren't even difficult plays. They were routine fly balls that dropped because you weren't there. We probably should've beaten that team. I don't know if it would have made a difference, but you had a chance to play, and you weren't ready, and that showed. At least to me, it showed. Every time you're out of position, it makes all of your jobs harder."

"I didn't think about it from a team perspective," admitted Ava. "My bad."

"That's why I'm saying something," said Zoe. "Look, I sometimes make physical mistakes and occasional errors. Those are understandable. However, mental mistakes are preventable and hurt our team. I try to prepare for every situation and look ahead for every play. I don't have your athleticism, but I would like to think quicker. If I can be prepared and be a step ahead of our opponents mentally, then I might be able to make up for my lack of athletic ability. I want to try to finish the year strong, and no way that will happen if we're unprepared. It's more important than ever now that Piper is hurt."

"I hear you. I just don't believe it's going to be worth it all the time. I'm not sure I want to take the time to prepare and then not play."

"You might not be getting the chances you want from Coach. It also might not be worth it from your perspective. But if you aren't prepared and fail when given the opportunity, do you think you'll get that chance again?" asked Zoe.

Zoe, Ava thought silently, in some ways, I hope you're done lecturing me. I know I can be stubborn. But I've always envied your perspective on things. And I know you're right.

Zoe continued, "You'll probably prove that Coach is right by not playing you. I know that you don't like that you aren't playing, and that leads you to not care, but it becomes a vicious cycle that hurts you and the team. You're mad you aren't playing, so you choose not to prepare. Then you finally get a chance but aren't prepared, so you do poorly. This causes Coach not to play you anymore, and then you'll have a bad attitude again."

"Thanks, Socrates!" joked Ava. "I can tell you're paying attention in your Intro to Philosophy course."

"Now that you mention it, I'm reminded of one of my favorite philosophers and literary scholars."

"Oh, yeah? Who's that?" inquired Ava.

"Captain Jack Sparrow from Pirates of the Caribbean, of course," said Zoe, smirking. "Captain Jack said that the problem is not the problem but that the problem is your attitude toward the problem."

"Deep. Real deep."

"Make jokes all you want. It's true," Zoe responded. "Not playing stinks. But you still get opportunities once in a while. The real problem is your attitude toward not playing. That leads you not to be prepared. If tonight was a really close game and you got to play, you could have been the X-factor one way or another. You would have played poorly because of being unprepared, which could have kept us from winning a close game. On the flip side, think if you had been prepared and were called into action in a close game. Combine your preparation with your athletic ability; you could have been the difference maker and helped propel us to victory."

"But it wasn't a close game."

"Absolutely, but you don't always know the situation. You have to train and prepare for when your opportunity comes. Don't worry about the situation. Just be prepared. If you had been prepared tonight, we probably wouldn't have won because it had such a large margin, but remember, we came back twice last year from bigger margins against better teams, so you never really know."

"I guess so," Ava said somewhat dismissively.

"You guess so, but I know so! It reminds me of what the Navy SEALs say."

"I know, I know," Ava interrupted. "'The only easy day was yesterday.'"

"Well, that is a great quote, but it wasn't what I was going to say."

"By all means, continue, ole wise one!" joked Ava.

"I thought of another one just now as you were mocking me. The Navy SEALs say, *The more you sweat in training, the less you bleed in battle*, but that wasn't what I originally thought about. The one I really like is 'Under pressure, you don't rise to the occasion but instead sink to the level of your training.'"

"I guess those make sense."

"You bet they make sense," said Zoe. "Today, you had the opportunity to play. But, no matter how badly you may have wanted to do well, you wouldn't be your best. More importantly, you weren't going to be what our team needed. You could have tried to rise to the occasion, but it wouldn't matter if you hadn't been ready. You didn't have it in you to be your best. You couldn't rise to the occasion because you hadn't prepared."

Ava thought about this moment like a lightbulb had come on above her head.

"My grandpa used to say something weird that I just thought about as you were talking. He used an Abe Lincoln quote. I guess honest Abe would say that if he had six hours to cut down a tree, he'd spend the first four hours sharpening the blade."

"That's cool. I hadn't heard that one before," said Zoe. "I do remember the quote by Benjamin Franklin when he said *by failing to prepare, you're preparing to fail.* If everyone on our team did a little more of that, we'd be ready for our opportunities when they come our way."

"I wonder if this place has one of those power banks? I should be prepared," Ava said.

Just then, Mr. Frank approached the two players as they were talking.

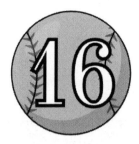

OPPORTUNITY KNOCKS

M r. Frank had refilled his coffee tumbler when he saw the two roommates talking. He was always impressed by how Zoe and Ava could be very different from one another but still demonstrate mutual respect. Though they had only been roommates since the beginning of the school year, they had a special friendship that allowed for some tough conversations, much like Haley and Kylee.

"I couldn't help but hear some of your ladies' conversation," he said. "You know, I've found that for much of my life, the harder I prepared, the luckier I seemed to get. I think that success can occur when opportunity meets preparation. Sure, there are times when we prepare, and that opportunity we so desperately want never actually comes to us. But I'd much rather be prepared, just in case. I'm not sure I'd want to live with the regret of knowing that something was right there before me, but I wasn't ready."

Neither of the players could argue with that. It made sense to both of them.

"This might seem like a silly question, but have you ever seen the movie *Titanic*?" Mr. Frank asked.

"Yes, but it's been awhile," said Zoe.

"My mom talks about it quite often," said Ava. "That was the movie they saw on their first date. Evidently, she had a crush on the guy in the movie but still was able to convince my dad to go see it with her."

"Well, I'm glad it worked out for them," said Mr. Frank. "Interestingly enough, Leonardo DiCaprio was not the director's first choice to play the lead role of Jack Dawson. He wasn't even the second, third, or fourth choice."

"How can that be true?" asked Ava. "I thought he was a super star. I thought he was popular."

"He wasn't a huge star then," replied Mr. Frank. "When he was younger, he had done a few commercials, some television shows, and a few films. But he hadn't yet become an international star. They considered the role of Jack Dawson for a few unknown actors you've never heard of and a few you probably have, like Tom Cruise."

"Once again, I feel some lesson coming from you, Mr. Frank. I'm guessing Leo was either really prepared or at the right place at the right time," Zoe said.

"Oh, Leonardo was prepared and definitely in the right place for his big break. But, if it weren't for the director taking a chance on an actor who wasn't yet a superstar, *Titanic* wouldn't have been the highest-grossing movie of all time."

"Sounds like the guy that took advantage of his opportunity," said Zoe.

"That's right. Leo was more than ready for his chance. I know that's a story about a movie star, but it happens in athletics all the time. A New England Patriots quarterback named Drew Bledsoe got hurt in a game and lost his job to a guy who was the 199th pick in the NFL draft. That guy was Tom Brady. Quarterback of the St. Louis Rams Trent Green got hurt in a preseason game and was replaced by a guy who had been stocking shelves at a grocery store for $5.50 an hour. That guy was Kurt Warner. Warner won the Super Bowl and was an eventual Hall of Famer. Green Bay Packers quarterback Don Majkowski broke his ankle in a game and was replaced by a guy named Brett Favre. Favre played the next 253 consecutive games for the Packers, which is an NFL record. He would win a Super Bowl and earn his way into the Hall of Fame.

"Mr. Frank, you really like football, don't you?" asked Ava. "It seems you're always talking about football."

"Sure do. I played a little halfback myself in college. I like to use football stories and analogies, but you can find many stories about players who got a chance and weren't ready. The sad reality is you don't usually hear about them. You look back and wonder why such and such team didn't fulfill its potential. Since you ladies are softball players, here's a softball story that just came to my mind."

As a deep thinker and a philosophy major, Zoe loved to hear good stories. Maybe, more importantly, she was excited because she hoped Mr. Frank would deliver a lesson that would speak to her roommate, Ava, and go along with what Zoe had been trying to tell her.

"I really enjoy watching the College World Series, as I'm sure you do," began Mr. Frank. "I'm sure you ladies know Montana Fouts, the pitcher from Alabama."

"Know her?" Zoe asked sarcastically. "Libby idolizes her. Montana was amazing. She won like a zillion pitching awards."

"During the SEC tournament her senior year, she landed wrong on her knee and was injured," continued Mr. Frank. "As it turns out, it was an ACL tear. But they didn't know it then. Regardless, Fouts couldn't pitch, and they had the NCAA Regional coming up. People wrote off Alabama when Fouts got injured. People feared there was no way they could make a run in the NCAA tournament without her. A young lady named Jaala Torrence, who had pitched very little that season, stepped in, put the team on her shoulders, and led the Crimson Tide into the NCAA Tournament. Jaala basically said, 'Give me the ball, and let's go'. They didn't win the National Championship that year, but that is not the point. Jaala was physically and mentally prepared when her time came."

"That is amazing," said Ava. "I didn't know that."

"Many people loved that story because neither Montana nor Jaala cared who got the credit. They just wanted to win. Montana was like a big sister to Jaala. They had each other's backs. The reason I tell you ladies that story is because the coach would say later that Jaala was mentally as tough as they come. That only comes through preparation. Jaala was called upon to take over for Montana when they needed her, and she was ready."

There it was. That was the lesson Zoe had been hoping for. It seemed that Ava was listening intently to Mr. Frank's story. It had to have touched a nerve.

"Thanks for sharing, Mr. Frank. I probably need to prepare myself better, especially if my goal is to help my team win," Ava said with a big grin.

"Yeah, thanks, Mr. Frank," Zoe added.

"You're very welcome, ladies. Just remember that everybody wants to be a champion. With all that said, hopefully, your cell phones are charged because it's about time to get back on the road. As the Bandit says, 'We've got a long way to go and a short time to get there.'"

"The Bandit?" asked Ava as she checked how much charge her phone now had.

"You know, Burt Reynolds from *Smokey and the Bandit*. It's a classic. My grandson absolutely loves it, but we have to keep telling him that it's not good to run from the cops, even though Burt Reynolds looks cool doing it. We have to remind my grandson it's just a movie. It's just entertainment. Anyway, I know you don't care about all of that or an old movie, so we probably need to get loaded up."

They watched Mr. Frank walk out the door.

"That Mr. Frank is wise," Zoe pointed out.

'Yeah, but ancient," added Ava. "I never heard of that movie."

"He might be ancient, but we're young. We don't know it all."

"Wait, what?!?" said a smiling Ava.

"We don't know it all, but I get the sneaky suspicion we might start knowing more. The more we prepare, the more we'll know, which might give us the edge we need."

"I'm going to use the bathroom, get a drink, and then meet you on the bus, but I want to let you know you've inspired me. That is, you and Mr. Frank. And now I'm convinced I must be prepared. I need to be ready. When opportunity knocks, I need to be ready to answer the door."

"That's awesome to hear," Zoe responded. "But remember Coach's rule about the buddy system. I'll go with you. Now, let's hurry up so we get on the bus before Libby and Gretchen!"

DR. EVAN'S CLASS

It hadn't been long since the team had been at the travel center. Normally, after a pit stop like that, everyone is wide awake and talkative. Tonight was no exception, but some of the players had tests coming up that they needed to prepare for.

"Hey, Haley, are you going to play cards with us in a few minutes?" asked Brooklyn.

"I don't think I'll be able to, thanks. I have a bunch of homework to get done."

"Oh, my goodness, what a nerd!" Brooklyn joked.

"Facts. Probably one of us should see an 'A' at some point in our lives," Haley snapped back. "Be nice to nerds. You'll most likely work for one someday."

"Okay, okay, haha, everyone's a comedian. You know this college thing wouldn't be so bad if we didn't have to go to class."

"99% of college is being committed enough to go to class," replied Haley. "Skipping class is the worst thing we can do. Being lazy and staying in bed is free. And, you know what my man Ed Sheeran said: 'The worst things in life come free to us.'"

At this point, Haley's roommate Megan decided to chime in and get in on the banter.

"Or, as my girl Taylor Swift says: 'In life, you learn lessons. And sometimes you learn them the hard way. Sometimes you learn them too late,'" Megan said.

Even though Megan was a year behind Haley in school, they had roomed together ever since Haley hosted Megan on a recruiting visit. Megan had been a solid player so far in her three years with the Eagles. She was well-liked and had a good sense of humor. She would be a fine captain next year when she was a senior and her roommate had graduated.

"Seriously though, you know I'm not much for school, but Dr. Evans's class is my favorite," said Brooklyn. "When I was in elementary school, my dad would pick me up, and he'd ask me what my favorite thing was about the day, and I would always say recess. Well, not always. Sometimes, I would say music or art."

"That's deep. Thanks so much for sharing something so personal," Megan snarked.

"Anyway, like I was saying. Dr. Evans is cool, and his class is tolerable," continued Brooklyn.

"Tolerable? That's some high praise coming from you," said Megan.

"It is what it is."

Dr. Daniel Evans was a trendy teacher at their school. He taught an odd combination of History and sports management classes and had a special way of connecting with the students and making his material relevant. Not only did he teach about the world of sports, but he also tried to tie it in with life through history. Many of the athletes liked taking his classes because he wasn't boring and kept them engaged. He sometimes even played his guitar for his students.

"Do you remember last week in class when we were talking about facilities and getting stadiums and arenas ready for games?" asked Megan. "It's crazy how quickly they can transform an ice hockey rink into a basketball court and all that goes into getting the grass and the field ready for baseball and football games when those teams have grass," said Megan.

Brooklyn added, "What stood out to me was the fact that nobody ever knows who those people are. They also get paid very little, relatively speaking, and yet they have some of the most important jobs of anyone in the organization in order for that game to be played. I know you need players to play a game, but those millionaires don't play if the field or court isn't ready."

"I liked the field trip he took us on last week," said Megan. "It was awesome to see how it all works for a professional baseball organization."

"That was awesome," agreed Brooklyn. "Were you as surprised as I was in how much pride those people had in working for that organization? Even though they were getting paid nothing compared to their bosses sitting at desks or the players, they still enjoyed their work and knew that it mattered."

"That was a little unexpected," said Megan.

"After that field trip, Dr. Evans actually brought that up to some of us. He said they were constantly reminding themselves of how important their work was. They worked as a team to make the game possible for the real team that everybody knows."

Megan nodded her head in agreement, saying, "It was funny how we were supposed to be learning about the nuts and bolts of operating a facility, and yet Dr. Evans found a way to talk about life and team and all that stuff."

"He even told that story about the Band of Brothers. Mr. Frank probably knows the story since he's so passionate about history," said Brooklyn.

Despite her efforts to do her homework, Haley was still half-listening to their conversation. Although she had never had Dr. Evans for a class, she had heard he was a good teacher.

"My uncle is an Air Force pilot right now, and his dad was retired from the Air Force," said Haley. "I love hearing their stories. What was the story Dr. Evans told you guys in class?"

"The Band of Brothers was about these paratroopers during World War II," Brooklyn told her. "While they were fighting in Belgium, the company inherited an incompetent commanding officer. Instead of commanding the group, the CO would go off and hide. The company had no leadership. So, a Staff Sergeant named Carwood Lipton would go around to every foxhole, check on the men, keep them focused, keep morale up, and hold the company together during one of the most dangerous battles of the war: The Battle of the Bulge."

"Hey, we learned about that battle in school!" said Haley.

"Yeah, they teach you about who won and who lost, but not the personal stories of heroism. Dr. Evans told us that even though Lipton's role was not what he had signed up for, he realized that his role had to change to one of leadership to save the men. He recognized the importance of having a leader the men could count on. If he hadn't accepted and excelled in his new role, many of the soldiers may have died. His role may have seemed minor then, but it was crucial to the company."

"Like my theater teacher my sophomore year always said, 'There are no small parts, only small actors,'" added Haley.

"That reminds me that I still have to take some kind of performing arts or music class," said Brooklyn. "I'm looking forward to that even though I wish I could just play softball all the time. But, I know that school is important. It's just hard to get out of bed some days."

"Or go to recess all the time," Megan said with a smile.

"At least I know you were listening to me," said Brooklyn.

"That Lipton story was interesting to me," said Megan. "I'm glad Dr. Evans shared it with us. He said that on all teams, whether in sports, a family, in business, or in the military, what one person does affects everybody else. That company's CO's lack of leadership could have killed everyone in the company. He said that bad leaders don't make bad decisions. Bad leaders make no decisions. He also said that most people think the term 'role player' is a dirty phrase. But it's just a matter of perspective. A role player is just someone playing a particular role, and roles frequently change. Caitlyn Clark can be a role player."

Megan could tell by Brooklyn's expression that she was a little confused about how a star like Caitlyn Clark could be a role player.

"On some plays, Caitlyn Clark is supposed to shoot. In some plays, she's supposed to set screens. On other plays, she might need to make passes. Her role depends on what the team needs," added Megan.

"But isn't being labeled a role player kind of degrading? It's like you don't have any talent," wondered Brooklyn.

"That isn't the way we should look at it," said Megan. "A role player has talent. Their talent is in the role they are playing. Lipton may not have officially had the title of leader. He may not have been the one most qualified to lead, but his talent ended up saving many lives. If we're a true team, then we want people who help, complement each other, and step up when needed. If you have a team full of selfish players, and no one is willing to do what it takes to win, the team will suffer."

"I guess it's all about your perspective," said Brooklyn.

"Role players need to be appreciated," said Megan. "The players who run bases for us in practice, for example. No one ever mentions them or how important they are to the success of the team. They may not get much playing time in games, but what they do to make the team better is crucial. Those roles need to be celebrated."

Megan nodded in agreement with Brooklyn's comment and then further explained her thoughts on roles.

"You're right, Brooklyn. If our perspective or focus is centered on us or on getting recognized in the newspaper or on TV, then we probably don't want to be known as a role player in a traditional sense. I'll tell you what, though, being a role player is extremely valuable to the team. If I'm a star, I want people around me willing to embrace their roles and be a star in their roles. If I were a pitcher instead of a first baseman, I would treat my fielders well, especially my catcher. I want my fielders to believe in me, dive for balls, and have my back if I make a bad pitch. I want my catcher blocking balls, framing pitches, and stealing strikes. We're all in this together. If we're not all doing our jobs, then we don't all experience success. In basketball, I once heard it said that it takes ten hands to make a basket. Everybody on the court or on the field has to believe in each other and help one another out."

"I never really thought about that from either perspective. I've always just figured stars are stars, and everyone else is just a role player," said Brooklyn.

"Right, but 'just a role player,' as you say, can mean so many things," said Megan. "Remember that a star can be a role player in a particular play. Like I said earlier, even Caitlyn Clark might have to pass or screen on a play. If she acts like a prima donna or doesn't want to star in this so-called lesser role, that could hurt her team. It could also cost her a chance to accomplish her goal of winning a championship."

Despite needing to study, Haley was having trouble concentrating on her work. The conversation between Megan and Brooklyn interested the Senior co-captain, as she thought of a story that would fit right into what they were talking about regarding player roles.

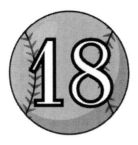

MOST VALUABLE TEAMMATE

Haley re-entered Brooklyn and Megan's conversation. She had a story of her own that would highlight the importance of all roles on a team.

"I played basketball with a girl named Carly back in high school. Though she was talented, she wasn't the star scorer. Her role was a practice player. In practice, she would play the role of small forward on the scout team and took her job very seriously. She studied film on the opponent and did her best to mimic the play of the other team's small forward in practice. Although we won back-to-back state championships with her on the team, she never played a minute of any tournament game. We all voted Carly as our Most Valuable Teammate."

"That's a cool story. I never knew that," said her roommate, Megan.

"But that's not the whole story," Haley continued. "Carly graduated early from college last spring with honors. On a whim, she sent a resume to an enormous and very popular computer company on the West Coast. Sure enough, the company called her and asked her for an interview.

"Wow, that's even cooler!" Brooklyn agreed.

Haley continued. "During the interview, they asked her, 'Carly, I see that you played on two state championship teams in high school. How many points did you score? What awards did you receive?' Carly replied, 'No. No. That wasn't my role on those teams. My role was to play the other team's small forward in practice. It was important to my team that I make our starting five better. I didn't play in either of the state championship games.'"

"So, she didn't get the job then because she wasn't the star?" asked Megan.

"She was hired right then and right there by one of the largest computer companies in the world," Haley said. "You see, big companies are just like teams. They want people who understand their roles and are willing to do whatever it takes to have the team win. Carly played her role, and we were all champions."

"That's amazing," said Brooklyn.

"Unfortunately, I played with another girl who missed out on some big-time scholarships," said Haley. "This girl had some talent. But she wouldn't listen to anyone, including the coaches. She had a couple of flaws in her swing that were easily correctable. One day, one of the coaches was working with her on the tee to help keep her hands up. When the session was over, she came over to me and said, 'I don't care what our coach wants me to do. I'm going to do it my way.'"

"I know someone like that," Brooklyn said, shaking her head.

"That's not the worst of it," related Haley. "Not only was she not coachable, but she was also a terrible teammate. She'd trash the coaches when no one was around, and she would also trash other players on our team. During practice, she would chew out a teammate for a bad throw, but when she threw the ball away, she made some ridiculous excuse. The other girls really resented her."

Megan said, "I never realized how important being a good teammate really is."

"And nothing was ever her fault," Haley continued. "Whenever she missed the ball in the field, it was always because of a bad hop. If she struck out, it was always because of the umpire. If she got a bad grade in school, it was the teacher's fault. She never held herself accountable for anything. Her attitude was toxic."

"Excuses," said Brooklyn. It wasn't a question. It was a statement.

"Even worse, ladies, when she was being recruited, the college coaches who were following her found out she was a below-average student. As soon as the coaches discovered that, no college would touch her. The reality is that thousands of athletes with similar skill sets work hard in and out of school and are good teammates."

"Stinks to be her," Megan said.

"Yes, but it also stunk to be her teammate," said Haley. We wondered how much better we could've been and how many more games we might've won if she'd been coachable and a great teammate," said Haley.

"I would have hated to play on a team with her," Brooklyn said. "I hate it when people make lame excuses for themselves."

"It was tough, Brooklyn," Haley said. "It was even tougher on the younger players on that team that looked up to her. Younger players look to the older players to see how to behave. Some of the younger players started to do the same things she did. That's what happens when you have a toxic player on your team."

"I know someone like that, too," Brooklyn commented.

Even though she should've been focusing more on her homework, Haley continued to enjoy the conversation. Brooklyn needed to hear this since she'd been struggling with her commitment to the team. Brooklyn was not a starter or every-day player. When she got the chance to play it was normally as a pinch hitter or to play the occasional inning in the outfield.

"When I hear that story, I think of the Navy SEALs," said Megan. "Haley, I know that you have family in the military. You know what kind of training they have to go through?"

"Some of it is insane," Haley remarked.

"During training, all the SEALs students are broken down into boat crews," Megan began. "Each crew is seven students, three on each side of a small rubber boat and one coxswain to help guide the dingy. Every day, the boat crew forms up on the beach and is instructed to get through the surf zone and paddle several miles down the coast. In the winter, the surf off San Diego can get to be eight to ten feet high, and it isn't easy to paddle through the plunging surf unless everyone digs in. Every paddle must be synchronized to the stroke count of the coxswain. Everyone must exert equal effort, or the boat will turn against the wave and be dumped back on the beach. For the boat to make it to its destination, everyone must paddle."

"Megan, we have some people on this team who aren't paddling. In fact, I think what they are doing is actually drilling holes in the boat. What I'm realizing now is that if we want to be a successful team, we're going to need help from each other, including our coaches, families, and our leaders," commented Brooklyn.

"It's a great analogy," said Haley. "There are probably other stories like that. It's not just sports that requires great teammates to be successful."

Megan agreed with her roommate, "Yep. I imagine that the best teams in sports are made up of players who want to excel in their roles, regardless of what those roles are, just like Carly. The best teams help each other and pick up the slack for one another. The best teams don't care who gets the credit. They celebrate successes together. They overcome challenges together. They win and lose together. They make sure that all the jobs and roles are filled regardless of who has to do them."

"Dr. Evans would be proud that you guys talked about him and his class so much tonight," said Haley.

"Maybe this conversation could be extra credit," suggested Megan.

"I don't think that'll work, Megan," said Brooklyn with a smile. "But I think it is a good idea to get everyone on this team to start paddling."

MUDITA

The bus was equipped with plenty of large monitors, giving every player a premium view of whatever game was being broadcast.

Like many of her teammates, Brooklyn loved to watch all sports and was particularly excited about the international soccer game on the monitors. She provided nonstop chatter, which Libby and Gretchen couldn't avoid since they were sitting nearby.

"This game's been awesome," said Brooklyn. "It's been back and forth the whole time. I played a lot of club soccer when I was growing up. I kind of miss it."

"It's been fun to watch even though I'd preferred to have heard more of the announcers than you," Libby said to Brooklyn.

"What can I say? I get excited watching good soccer," Brooklyn said. "Soccer is one of those sports that shows the importance of everyone's teamwork. Only one person scores the goal, but everyone on the team plays a part in putting the ball in the back of the net. And everyone gets excited when someone scores."

Gretchen and Libby looked at each other and rolled their eyes.

Brooklyn continued to talk. "But, football season will be back at the end of the summer and then you'll get to listen to me drone on about my Super Bowl Champion Kansas City Chiefs."

"Yeah, I didn't watch much of that game," Libby said. "For me, I was only paying attention to 87 times they turned the camera on my girl Taylor Swift."

"I kind of like the Super Bowl party," Gretchen said. "The food is amazing. My mom loves the commercials."

"I bet there is something about my amazing Chiefs you didn't know," Brooklyn said.

"Okay, go ahead and tell us Patrick Mahomes is cuter than Tom Brady, blah, blah, blah," Libby retorted.

"Oh, no. None of that," Brooklyn replied. "My 2024 Super Bowl Champion Kansas City Chiefs didn't have a single 1000-yard rusher or 1000-yard receiver. In fact, neither did the 2019 Patriots nor the 2018 Eagles. None of them did. To top it off, the 2018 Eagles had a backup quarterback to lead them through the playoffs and to the championship."

Libby acknowledged the statistic. "Pretty impressive," she said.

Megan was almost as big a fan as Brooklyn, so she entered the conversation.

"I think Brooklyn is trying to make the point that the best teams aren't always made up of the best individual talent," Megan suggested. "Here is another statistic that will blow your mind. Michael Jordan won four NBA scoring titles before he won an NBA championship. Jordan could not do it himself, even with all that talent. And history is repeating itself with Luka Dončić of the Dallas Mavericks. He might be the best player in the NBA right now; he just won the scoring title. During the playoffs, he averaged nearly 30 points a game, 10 rebounds, and 10 assists, leading his team in every category. But his team almost got swept by the Boston Celtics in the finals."

"Megan, you sound like you're going to have a career in coaching someday," Brooklyn observed.

"Maybe so. But it reminds me of a post I saw on social media," related Megan. "It said, 'Every team in America has starters and a leading scorer. What does it matter if you're a starter or a star player? Not every team in America wins. Winning is more difficult and special than being a starter or star.'"

"Wow, that statement kind of punches you right between the eyes, huh?" Brooklyn said.

"That's probably how your beloved Chiefs went about their business, Brooklyn," said Megan. "We before me. I'm guessing that's not just a cliche for those guys."

"And Taylor Swift's beloved receiver Travis Kelce had his worst statistical season in almost 10 years. He didn't reach 1,000 receiving yards but they didn't need him to be a stat star. They needed him to be great teammate that did whatever the team needed. They valued team performance, instead," Brooklyn pointed out.

"Ladies, I get y'all are slow-walking us to some lightbulb moment," Libby stammered. "Can we get to the point? We're a softball team, not a soccer, football, or basketball team."

"Maybe we need to start approaching things like those Super Bowl Chiefs and not be concerned about who gets the credit or accolades," Megan suggested. "More to the point, we have to put our egos to the side and be concerned about the team. We play a team sport, after all."

"Hey, sorry to interrupt," said Brooklyn. "But there's a video my high school coach sent me. It's about being a great teammate. I think everyone should listen to this. I'll send it to you when I'm done."

One of the players asked Mr. Frank to turn off the TV so they could hear Brooklyn. All the players gathered around her. The only sound was the hum of the tires on the road.

"This story happened at the University of Alabama in 2009 at the College World Series," Brooklyn began. "Alabama was down 4-2 in the bottom of the 4th inning with two outs, the bases loaded, in an elimination game. Due up to the plate was Brittany Rogers. Brittany was a four-time All-American outfielder and a senior leader."

"Sounds like a great opportunity to be the hero," Libby said.

"But Coach Patrick Murphy took her out of the game and put in a freshman to hit for her."

"WHAT?!?" exclaimed Gretchen. "Murph took her out for a freshman? If this is an elimination game, that might be her last career at-bat!"

"That's right, Gretchen. But, before I continue with my story, you're a senior. What would YOU do if you were four-time All-American Brittany Rogers, and you got taken out?"

"I would be so pissed! I would probably go to the end of the dugout and pout," Gretchen related. "Maybe I would stick pins in my Coach Murphy doll."

"Well, that's not what Brittany did," Brooklyn continued. "Brittany became the biggest cheerleader at the very top of the dugout steps. Brittany's substitute was a girl named Jazlyn Lunceford. Jazlyn quickly got two strikes on her. But she showed incredible confidence at the plate. She managed to even the count to 2-2 and fouled off a couple more pitches. Like I said, Brittany was at the dugout's top step, cheering and screaming for Jazlyn. Jazlyn just kept fighting. The tension built in the at-bat. The game announcers discussed Coach Murphy's decision to replace the senior leader with a freshman. Finally, on the 6th pitch of the at-bat, Jazlyn smashed an opposite-field home run into the left-field stands."

"My skin is tingling!" Libby said.

"My heart is racing," freshman Zoe said.

"That's amazing!" said Gretchen. "Coach Murphy is a genius for putting her in the game!"

"That's not the amazing part," Brooklyn said. "Brittany Rogers was the first out of the dugout and the first to tackle Jazlyn at the plate when she crossed, jumping around like crazy."

Megan had a thought that she couldn't hold back. She looked her teammates in the eye. "I'm thinking, ladies, about what Gretchen said she might have done: go to the end of the dugout and pout. What do you think would have been going through Jazlyn's head if Brittany had done that: go and pout? 'Oh, Brittany is going to hate me!' or 'We're never going to be friends again!' Would she ever have hit that homerun?"

Silence. Just the hum of the bus tires.

"Instead, Brittany demonstrated 100% trust and confidence in her teammate," Brooklyn continued. "I found out later that before the at-bat, Brittany put her hands on Jazlyn's shoulders and said, 'You got this, Jaz.' She showed complete confidence in Jaz. She believed in her. She encouraged her even if Jaz was potentially taking her last career at-bat. Wait until you see this video. I've never seen an athlete so excited. And, she was excited about someone else hitting a home run!"

Mr. Frank was listening intently, proud of what he was hearing.

"'It's amazing what you can accomplish if you don't care who gets the credit,'" Mr. Frank said. "Harry S. Truman."

Several players had tears in their eyes.

"According to Coach Murphy, it's called Mudita," Brooklyn continued. "It means 'Vicarious joy in someone else's accomplishments' in Sanskrit. There's no word for it in the English language. Ladies, when we decide to be more excited about what someone else achieves than our selfish interests, we're going to have an amazing team. We have to start playing for each other, be genuinely excited for each other, and stop being so selfish. When I say *genuine*, I mean *genuine*. A 1st grader can tell when someone is not being real with them."

"Wow," Libby said quietly to herself. "You have given me a lot to think about. As one of your pitchers, I'm realizing that maybe I'm trying to do too much by trying to strike everyone out and get my numbers up. Maybe I should focus more on hitting spots and getting hitters to mis-hit balls and get more outs, as coach said."

"Yeah, and I've been striking out too much because I've been overswinging trying to hit bombs," Gretchen added.

"And I was not ready when my time came today," Kylee added. "I let myself, my team, and my dad down."

Piper, who had been listening quietly, finally spoke. "Ladies, our coaches love us and want the best for us. Sure, they get upset sometimes because we're not meeting our standards and aren't doing things that are in the team's best interest. We can't have a bunch of players with their own personal agendas, like Libby and Gretchen said. We all need to love, support, and encourage each other. We can't let each other down. Each of us must live up to the standards we set for ourselves. We need to make the decision that *this is the way we do things here.*"

Megan said, "I think it's a good idea that we all look at ourselves in the mirror. None of us wants to be selfish, as Libby mentioned a few minutes ago."

Brooklyn said, "I like those thoughts, Megan. Just like my beloved Kansas City Chiefs. 'We before me.' Maybe we can become like that."

"You may be on to something here," Libby said, acknowledging Megan's observation.

"Exactly," said Megan. "We all want to be part of a great team, but a great team requires great teammates. Are we those people on this team? We won't have a championship team if we don't encourage, support, and have each other's backs."

"I have an idea," freshman Zoe announced. She stood up from her seat.

"What's up, freshie?" Libby asked.

"I know I'm only a freshman," Zoe said. "But I'm going up to the coach's seat and ask him if we can have 'Mudita' stickers made that we can put on the back of our batting helmets. It would be a constant reminder for us to be great teammates."

Megan rose and put both hands on Zoe's shoulders. "You got this, Zoe," she said.

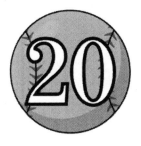

THE DREAM TEAM

Brooklyn had finished with her story and shared the video with all of her teammates. Some of the Eagles still couldn't believe the incredible story—not of the homerun but of the unselfishness Brittany Rogers displayed.

The Eagles still had some time left on their trip. Satellite TV still offered many entertainment options for those not on Snap or TikTok or deep in thought.

"Hey, Coach. Please keep it on this channel," Gretchen asked. "The documentary about the Dream Team is coming up next."

"My dad said that was the best basketball team ever," said Libby. "I guess it was the first time they ever let professionals play. Before that, you had to be an amateur to play."

"That's right," said Coach Batdorff. "Some people say The Dream Team was the best sports team ever assembled. That team had 11 future NBA Hall of Famers on it, including Michael Jordan, Magic Johnson, and Larry Bird. And, they only had one rule: Be on time."

Libby and Gretchen shared a sly smile with each other.

"They went undefeated in the 1992 Olympics, right?" asked Gretchen.

"Not only did they go undefeated, but they won all their games by an average of 44 points." Coach Batdorff said. "But, their influence transcended the game of basketball."

"What do you mean 'transcended,' Coach?" Gretchen asked.

"By The Dream Team winning the gold medal in basketball at the 1992 Olympics, thousands or perhaps millions of young people picked up basketballs," Coach Batdorff related. "The sport of basketball took off even more after that. The league expanded again, adding two teams in Canada. The Dream Team did more than win a gold medal. They inspired millions of kids to be just like them. It was essentially a rebirth of the sport. Millions of athletes today owe their interest in basketball to The Dream Team."

Brooklyn couldn't resist. "Coach, you want to talk about a team that transcended their sport. How about the 1999 Women's World Cup Team?"

"Brooklyn, you're the soccer expert here," Coach Batdorff said with a smile.

"What the Women's World Cup team did changed women's sports forever," Brooklyn began. "Or, as President Clinton said, 'Changed the face of women's sport forever.' Not only did Brandi Chastain take her shirt off on national TV, with the whole world watching after scoring the winning goal on a penalty kick, but the team also inspired millions of kids, especially girls, to start kicking a soccer ball. Before the '99ers', as we say, you can argue that women's sports were not taken very seriously. Much of the success in women's sports today, locally, collegiately, and professionally, can be tied to what Mia Hamm, Carla Overbeck, and the others did."

"And then, there is the 1980 men's Olympic Hockey Team," Mr. Frank said from his driver's seat. "Now, you all weren't born; I was just a little kid. But no team in the history of American sports had a greater impact on American culture than that gold medal team."

"Oh, I love hockey," Zoe said. "I saw that movie. It's called Miracle."

"Well, Zoe, this is not really about hockey," Mr. Frank said. "Unlike the basketball Dream Team and the '99ers', this is not really about the sport. Yet, their influence changed the world."

Zoe squinted her eyes in confusion.

"In 1980, America didn't feel very good about itself. We had an oil crisis. We had American hostages in Iran. We were in the heart of the Cold War and arms race with the Soviet Union. The United States boycotted the Summer Olympics that year because it was held in Moscow. Americans didn't have a lot to cheer for. But, the Winter Olympics were held in Lake Placid, New York. The men's hockey team was comprised mostly of college kids from Boston and Minnesota. The Americans were fortunate enough to make it to the medal round but had to play the Russians in the semi-finals to make it to the gold medal game.

"A few weeks earlier, the same Russian team had played an exhibition game against a group of NHL all-stars, and the Russians beat them easily. So, obviously, no one gave the American college kids a chance. So much so that the USA v. Soviet Union game was not even on live television. It was taped-delayed. I remember watching, though. I remember the chants of 'USA, USA, USA' as time ticked by. The Americans scored some incredible goals and shut down the powerful Russian offense. I will never forget Al Michaels counting down '11 seconds, 10 seconds' and finally, 'Do you believe in miracles? Yes!'"

"But that wasn't even the gold medal game," Zoe said. "They had to play and beat Finland to win the gold."

"That's right, Zoe," Mr. Frank said. "And that's what they did. It was an incredible moment."

"But, Mr. Frank, you said it wasn't about the sport," Gretchen asked. "What do you mean?"

"Because the US had beaten the Russians in something, it gave America hope in everything," Mr. Frank said. "There was a rebirth in American patriotism. America started to believe in itself again.

America had a sense of pride again. We got our hostages back, unemployment decreased, and people purchased American-made products. It felt good to be an American again."

Piper, the injured centerfielder, had ice on her knee and was taking it all in. "Ladies, sometimes I think we lose sight of our influence on other people even if we're only a college softball team. We're extremely fortunate to be able to play this game. But the game is bigger than us, and we should be grateful for being able to play. You see the little girls who come to our games. They want to be like us. We need to be conscious of how influential we are. Just like The Dream Team, the 99ers, and the US hockey team."

"*Little Eyes Upon You*," said shortstop Haley. "It's a poem about how much we influence young people."

"I would like to make a suggestion to the team," Piper said, ice on her knee. "We should give back to this game that has been so good to us."

"How do we do that?" Libby asked. "All of us are super busy. And Brooklyn needs to get her grades up."

"By doing a softball camp for kids," Piper replied. "By having Gretchen showing kids how to be a catcher, by having Libby do a pitching clinic for little girls, by having Ava work with young outfielders, by having Kylee work with young hitters. And, everyone can help out with their position groups."

"I love that idea, Piper," said Megan. "Let's do it!"

"I will talk to Coach about it when we get back," Piper said. "Serving our sport and our community is one thing, and I'm all for it, but we also need to be better at leading ourselves. The 'little eyes that are on us' as Haley said. Kids will do exactly what we do. So, from here on out, we must commit ourselves to leading by example. We need to understand that what one of us does affects all of us."

Piper paused, and then said with a slight grin, "And we can start by everyone being on time."

Piper looked at Gretchen and Libby.

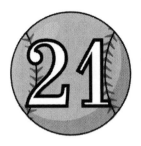

BACK AT SCHOOL

Libby couldn't help but smile at Piper's last comment.

"I don't know if she's being serious, but Piper does make a decent point," admitted Libby. "We're always late, and that probably isn't fair to the rest of the team."

"You're right, Libby," said Gretchen. "It's never been anything I've thought about, but it was important enough of a rule to be the only rule on The Dream Team. Their coach said they did it because it was more than being late for a bus or a team meal. It was about respect. It was a sign that the person didn't think they were better than someone else. I never thought about it that way."

Brooklyn mentioned, "Like this morning when you guys stopped to get fancy coffee and were late getting on the bus."

"There was a line at the coffee house," justified Libby. "And, like I told coach earlier, the coffee at the dorm is disgusting."

"You're not kidding," echoed Gretchen. "And you know the phrase, 'People with no decision-making ability can make six decisions to buy one cup of coffee: Short, tall, light, dark, caf, decaf, low-fat, non-fat, etc.'"

"That's right!" said Libby.

"What? I don't even know what you're talking about right now," Brooklyn said, shaking her head.

"It's from *You've Got Mail*. You know, that old rom com with Tom Hanks and Meg Ryan?" said Gretchen. "Forget about it. It doesn't matter. Anyway, we're coffee snobs and proud of it. But I think I get your point. We made the whole team late. At the very least, we weren't very respectful of everyone else's time."

"But, that coffee hit the spot," Libby pointed out again.

Brooklyn was starting to get a little frustrated, but it might have been because she was jealous that she didn't get one of those fancy drinks this morning.

"Okay, got it. The coffee was good. Coffee stains your teeth and gives you coffee breath," Brooklyn concluded. "Hey, Gretchen. How about the next game, you and Libby battle each other out and see who is more competitive? See which of you can win that contest. See which of you can get here first."

Piper adjusted the ice on her knee. "Being late is a choice, ladies," she said.

The bus started to slow down, and Kylee looked out the window at the sign for their exit.

"That's a sight for sore eyes," said Kylee.

"Almost there. Can't wait for my head to hit that bed," said Haley.

"No kidding," Kylee said. "I only have one class tomorrow. I'm not going to lie, I'm pretty tired. I'm not entirely disappointed we don't have practice tomorrow."

"I agree. It was pretty obvious that Coach didn't want to see us much tomorrow," Haley stated.

"He was a little frustrated with us, wasn't he?"

Kylee then continued with a thought, "I've been thinking about something ever since we talked earlier."

"What's that?" Haley asked.

"I think what you and I talked about would be good for everyone to hear," suggested Kylee. "Even though we aren't having practice, I think we should get everyone together tomorrow."

"A team meeting?" Haley asked.

"A team meeting," Kylee said. "But not one of those players-only ones where everyone moans and complains. What we talked about is pretty important. It could spur something on in other people's minds, as well. I mean, if it got me thinking, maybe it will get others thinking."

Haley agreed, "That's a good idea. I'll text everyone right now."

Dings and beeps could be heard across the bus as Haley's text message was delivered to her teammates' phones.

"That's weird," murmured Haley, looking at her phone.

"What's that?"

"Everyone responded," said Haley.

"Even Gretchen and Libby?" asked Kylee.

"Yes, even the dynamic duo. But that isn't what's weird," said Haley. "Not only did everyone respond, but nobody complained even though we were supposed to have the day off. That's the unusual part."

"Cool. Guess I can't take as long of an afternoon nap tomorrow as I was hoping," Kylee said.

"Nope, but your idea of a meeting will be a good thing. I think it will be better in the long run than your nap."

The players felt the bus come to a stop in the parking lot outside the practice field.

"Rise and shine, Cinderellas. Your chariot has arrived back at the castle," announced Mr. Frank.

"Your what and where?" said Kylee.

"That's just Mr. Frank," Haley said. "I'm not sure what he's saying sometimes, but I guess I know what he means."

"Whatever. I'm just glad to be home. Let's get off this bus."

As the players cleaned up around their seats, picked up the trash, and gathered their things, Piper approached Coach Batdorff with a limp as she navigated the bus aisle with her crutches.

"Hey, Coach. I know today was rough," Piper said. "The whole season's been rough. But try and get some sleep tonight. I know you'll want to be up before the roosters tomorrow, but try to sleep in a little later than usual. You're no good to us if you're tired and worn down. Even though you canceled practice because you were frustrated with us, we can turn that into a positive. Some of us can use the time to study or rest up. The same goes for you. Rest up a little. Use tomorrow to refresh yourself, and let's get back to it the day after."

"I appreciate that," Coach Batdorff said. "I'll see what I can do."

"Also, just to keep you in the loop. We're having a team meeting tomorrow. It's supposed to be a good team meeting. I'll personally make sure we stay focused on the positive stuff. I know that you've put a lot of trust in me over the years. I appreciate that. Trust me on this also, Coach."

"Thanks for letting me know."

"I know player-only meetings are often not very productive, but I was talking with Haley, and she assured me that this will be a positive thing and not like those meetings we hear about when a team rebels against a coach," Piper said reassuringly.

"Okay. Thanks again, Piper. Have a good night."

Piper left the bus with Jasmine right behind. Jasmine was another freshman on the team. She roomed with Tracy. The two of them respected Piper a great deal. Jasmine and Piper had a class together right before lunch and often got a bite to eat together.

"Hey, Piper, I just heard you talking with Coach about the meeting tomorrow. You also told him to get some rest and all that other stuff. That was different since you're a player, and he's a coach. I don't know if I noticed that before. It was almost like you were coaching him."

"Not coaching. Just encouraging," Piper replied. "I know early on in my softball career, I'd get mad with the coaches, teachers, or even my parents. They wouldn't encourage or praise me. About midway through my freshman year, I decided that instead of getting frustrated when someone didn't acknowledge me or recognize me for something,

I was going to turn and flip the script. I decided I would encourage or praise somebody instead."

"You always seem like you've got an encouraging word for somebody when they are down. I can't imagine you not being an encourager."

"It's not that I wasn't encouraging people at all. I just wasn't doing it enough. I also found that I wasn't doing it when I was feeling down or frustrated, myself."

"You said it was your freshman year when this changed. Did you have some vision or something?" Jasmine asked with a smirk on her face.

"No visions or alien abductions. It was Psych class," Piper said. "The teacher was sharing about this guy, Karl Menninger, who had been on the cover of TIME Magazine or something like that. One day, he was speaking to a large college class, and somebody asked him what a person should do if they were depressed or troubled. The person asking the question assumed that this noted psychologist would mention some counseling or cutting-edge treatment. Instead, Menninger said, 'Board up the house, go across the street, find someone in need, and go help them.' When I heard that, I decided to start encouraging others more. The only way for me to beat despair or frustrations was through engagement. I had to get out of my little world. I had to stop being selfish and encourage others. If I felt like I wasn't getting the encouragement, recognition, or praise that I wanted, then I was going to make sure that somebody else didn't feel that way, too."

"I never thought about it quite like that before."

"I hadn't either," Piper said. "I also realized that not just my teammates need encouragement. But my teachers, parents, custodians, coaches, even Mr. Frank. All those people need a kind word, smile, or breath of fresh air blown into their lives occasionally."

"You might consider starting your own greeting card company," Jasmine suggested. "You've got some great insights and deep thoughts."

"Thanks for the encouragement, Jasmine. I appreciate it. You asked me about Coach to start with, and I wanted you to know that I'm not trying to kiss up to him. That's not my intention. I just try to encourage him whenever I can. And it's not hollow encouragement. It's not the fake stuff. It's not like, 'Hey, Coach, we all love you, so keep doing what you're doing.' That wouldn't benefit anyone."

Jasmine chuckled and nodded her head in agreement. "I hate it when people say, 'You can do it' or 'Let's go,' but those are very generic. That doesn't motivate me very much."

"You're right. We should be saying things that have substance," Piper said. "We can always find something to encourage someone with. Even if one of my teammates is playing poorly, I can remind them of when they performed great. I can speak to the value they can bring to the team. I can remind them of all the preparation they put in."

As Piper was talking, Jasmine's eyes got huge as she remembered a situation from the previous week.

"Now that you say that, I remember last week when you said, 'Jasmine, you can do this. Let that riseball go. The best way to defeat the riseball is to not swing at it. The umpire will call it a ball anyway. Look for it down in the zone. And, when you get that ball down in the zone, don't miss it.' That motivated me because you put something real in my head. You didn't just say 'you can do it; you can do it' while clapping a lot."

Piper smiled at Jasmine's comment. "That's what I mean. We can always find some way to encourage others. I love it when others compliment or encourage me, so it has to work the same with others. If I can encourage others, they might be more motivated. If we're all doing that, then before you know it, maybe we have a team that's totally looking out for each other and lifting each other up. That goes for all of us, coaches, managers, support staff, and players. We're all in this together."

"Never thought of that," Jasmine said. "Thanks for sharing. See you tomorrow."

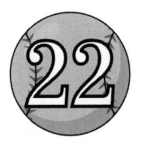

TEAM MEETING

As the players trickled in, the atmosphere was different. It wasn't depressing like the room usually was after a bad performance.

Gretchen and Libby were also among the first people there. That was remarkably strange but in a good way.

"Hey, Gretchen. Hey, Libby. Sorry about the mix-up in time," said Haley.

"What do you mean?" asked Gretchen.

"Well, you're here early. It's not 4:00 yet. You must have thought I said 3:30 or something like that."

"Haha, funny, Haley," said Libby. "We heard the right time. We're just here early."

"Cool. I'm just messing with you. We'll get started soon."

"That's fine. We were just a little inspired watching that documentary about The Dream Team last night," said Gretchen. "If it was good enough for the best team ever in the history of sports, then maybe we should be more respectful and start being on time."

"And, maybe one day Mr. Frank will be sick, and we'll have a substitute bus driver that leaves us behind," said Libby with a smile.

"I'm not sure a bus driver would leave a player behind, but maybe Coach would follow through on his threats," said Haley.

Almost in unison, Gretchen and Libby repeated the line that Coach Batdorff had often said, "My coach left me behind my senior year of college, and so any of you could get left behind, also."

"Regardless, though," said Haley. "You guys are saying things that are directly related to why Kylee and I wanted to have a team meeting today."

By now, all the players had arrived, so Kylee opened up the meeting.

"Haley and I were talking last night on the bus. I'm sure you all heard my dad got on Coach pretty hard after the game. That's how the conversation with Haley started. We've been friends for a long time, so she could say some things to me that if someone else had said them, I'm not sure I would have listened."

Kylee continued, "During our talk, I came to realize that I wasn't taking responsibility for my actions. I was making way too many excuses and not being focused. Because I'm a senior, I've been getting more and more frustrated about not playing. But this was leading me to act less and less as a senior leader should act. I realized I wasn't being the leader this team needed, whether I was playing or not. I wasn't setting a good example. I wasn't taking responsibility for my actions."

"Kylee's right," said Haley. "Our night started rocky with the poor performance in the game, and then her dad got up in Coach's face. But I think some good came from it. We might meet with the umpires before each game. We might have a 'C' next to our name on the roster. Our resume might say 'Captain.' Those things might be true, but we must be positive and effective leaders."

Eye contact, Haley. Look everyone in the eyes, she thought.

"Sure, Kylee has made excuses and not always acted like a captain, but we can all do better," continued Haley. "We can all take more responsibility for our actions. After all, we have a collective responsibility and are responsible for each other. Our actions and attitudes affect more than just us. As your leaders, we haven't done what we need to do. It starts with us. We have a position and maybe some status, but we haven't earned it day after day. We need to do a better job of helping this team be the best it can be. Not everything that happens is our fault just because we're captains. We may have a leadership position, but you need us to be good leaders. We need to earn your trust and respect. The title has to mean something."

The room was silent. Every eye was focused on Haley and Kylee as they spoke. What they were saying was a surprise, but it made sense in a weird way that the players had not previously thought about. As they processed their words, they realized that Kylee and Haley might be correct, but the team had confidence they would be the leaders they needed moving forward.

"Hey, ladies, thanks for sharing," Piper said. "I don't know about the rest of the team, but I believe in you and am glad that you're our captains. You guys are leaders, but it makes sense what you're saying. There's always room for improvement. Plus, we probably haven't been perfect followers, either. We all can do better."

"I agree with Piper," said Megan. "You guys are our captains for a reason. Whether or not you think you've done a good job doesn't matter right now. All that matters is that you want to get better, and that motivates me. I want to get better, too. If you think you can do better, we should all feel the same way and want to improve ourselves."

Megan continued, thinking, "What you're saying is interesting because Brooklyn and I had a conversation last night, too. We talked about starring in your role. About excelling in your role. When you're excellent in the role you have, everybody on the team benefits. Championship teams are made up of a bunch of stars. Not necessarily people in the spotlight but people excelling in their roles that complement one another. There were some things I hadn't really thought much about before. Talking with Brooklyn last night and then hearing you today makes me really want to try to be better and make this team better moving forward."

"When was the last time we appreciated and complimented our role players?" Brooklyn asked. "Take freshie, Zoe, for example. She runs the bases like crazy for us during practice. She makes the team better even though her name doesn't show up in the newspaper or even the box score. But what she does matters. We need to make sure what she does gets celebrated."

"Our bullpen catchers, too," said Gretchen. "I know I start most of the games at catcher and get a lot of the limelight. But Jasmine spends a lot of her time warming up my pitchers, and she is technically a backup outfielder. When was the last time you pitchers thanked Jasmine for what she does?"

Libby, Grace, and Tracy looked sheepishly at each other.

"Pitchers and catchers are a team-within-a-team," Grace said. "Libby, Tracy, and I appreciate our catchers even if we don't verbalize it. Catchers have to deal with us throwing balls in the dirt, and they are constantly bruised because of us. But good catchers steal strikes for us by framing pitches. I might get credit for the strikeout, but our catchers do a lot of the work. And, you're right, Gretchen, we need to do a better job and celebrate those roles."

"Here, Libby and I thought we were the ones trying to turn over a new leaf, start fresh, and begin living right," Gretchen said. "We thought we'd be the ones having to make changes through this conversation. Seriously, though, this is awesome. By the way, in case you didn't notice or hear me the first time, Libby and I were on time today."

"Actually, you were early," Kylee said.

"Anyway, we were early to this meeting because we realized last night that by being late to everything, we were essentially disrespecting all of you," said Gretchen. "We were saying that we were more important than you girls. We were acting all entitled and everything. We're sorry and will try to do better in the future. No guarantees that we'll always be early like today, but we should always be on time from here on out."

"Are you two making us a promise or a commitment?" Haley asked. "Promises and commitments are different things."

Libby and Gretchen looked at each other. "Commitment," both replied simultaneously.

"Gretchen is definitely speaking for me about this," echoed Libby. "But, listening to her talk, along with what Megan said and Haley and Kylee said, I think this meeting went a different direction than most of us probably expected after yesterday's game."

Just as remarkably as Gretchen and Libby showing up early to a meeting, heads seemed to be simultaneously nodding up and down around the room.

WHITEBOARD

The meeting had started unexpectedly, and the co-captains were determined to take advantage of the positive vibe from the rest of their team.

"Wow, I didn't expect this when we called this meeting," said Kylee. "I just wanted to apologize for being a bad leader and always making excuses. Haley and I wanted to let you know that we were going to do better, but it sounds like some of you also had productive conversations last night. If you guys don't mind, let's take a few more minutes and talk about these things. We can even act like Coach and write some stuff on the whiteboard to visualize it better."

Haley took her cue from Kylee, picked up the dry-erase marker, and approached the whiteboard. She erased a cross and crescent moon that had evidently been left by another group of students.

"Like Kylee and I said, we want to be more than captains. We want to be effective leaders. Like we talked about, we need to take more responsibility. Specifically, we need to stop making excuses. We could all stand to do better in this area at times, so I'm going to write down 'Lose the excuses.'"

After writing down 'Lose the excuses,' Haley continued. "Megan and Brooklyn, you talked about starring and excelling in your roles.

What if I put 'Excel in your role?' Does that sum up your conversation last night?"

"Yeah, that works," said Megan.

"And our *twins of promptness and punctuality* have finally seen the light and admitted that our time matters as well," joked Haley.

"Why don't you just write down 'Always be on time' and stop throwing shade," suggested Libby.

"Deal," said Haley. "So, we wrote three things up here. Does anyone have anything to add?"

"Thank you for giving everyone a voice, Haley," said Andrea. "But you made me feel guilty when we stopped in traffic forever after the game."

"It was only like 15 minutes, and if you felt guilty, it's because you had a guilty conscience already as opposed to it being something I said," replied Haley.

"Anyway, for those who didn't hear," continued Andrea. "She said that my attitude was like a flat tire, and I wouldn't get very far if I didn't fix it. I realized that I hadn't been displaying the best attitude. I guess I can be grumpy, and that doesn't spread enthusiasm or positivity. In fact, it can be quite contagious, like a sickness or something."

"Yeah, we don't want you to be a bacteria," joked Haley.

"She's right," added Piper. "We want you to be a big dose of Vitamin C, or D, or E, or whatever that thing is in orange juice that's supposed to make us healthy."

"Anyway. No, I don't want to be a bacteria, virus, or whatever. I need to show a good attitude and control my emotions," agreed Andrea.

"I think that's something we all should be doing, so I will add 'Display a good attitude' to the board. Thanks for sharing," said Haley.

After writing on the board, Haley looked at Jasmine, who was raising her hand and smiled.

"Hey, Jasmine. You don't have to raise your hand to speak. This isn't class or anything like that. If you have something to say, just speak up and say it."

"Sorry. Habit," said the freshman. "Anyway, I'm sure you've noticed, but Piper always has a really good attitude. She's always encouraging people."

The teammates nodded their heads in approval.

"Yeah, you probably knew that. But what you may not have seen her do, which I was able to witness, is how she encouraged Coach last night. Come to find out that she does that frequently. I know she has encouraged me throughout the year. Based on the looks on your faces, you agree with me. But it goes further. She encourages more than just her fellow teammates. She encourages everyone," said Jasmine.

"You're right, Jasmine," Haley confirmed. "Piper is quick with a compliment or praise. She always tries to be positive. She's encouraged me a bunch through the years. It's no surprise she encourages everybody in our program, not just her teammates. We're all a family. We're one program. I'm going to put what you said on the board."

Haley then wrote 'Encourage team members' on the whiteboard.

"I put team members instead of teammates because we should also strive to encourage managers, trainers, bus drivers, coaches, whoever. We're all in this together."

"Hey, Haley."

Haley looked at Libby, half expecting her to pat herself on the back again for honoring her commitment of being on time, but that wasn't why Libby was speaking up.

"Mr. Frank's story about those rugby players stuck on the mountain really spoke to me. I also liked hearing about that explorer guy."

"Cortez," interrupted Zoe, trying to help Libby.

"Yeah, thanks, freshie," replied Libby. "Anyway, I realized I probably wasn't very committed to this team, the process, or the journey if I was getting frustrated too easily and always losing focus.

It's been about me way too much, especially when I'm not making good pitches and walking people, like last night. I get rattled and doubt myself when this happens, so I'm probably not good to anyone. I don't think I've been committed to the team or focused very well lately, which I'm going to work on."

"Along with our commitment to being on time," Gretchen reminded her.

"Great point, both of you," said Haley. "Libby, I agree with what you're saying, but it isn't just you. I hadn't heard of either of those stories before Mr. Frank and Coach told them to us. But they speak to me, too. We thought we would be good this year for a bunch of different reasons, but we have played below our talent level. But maybe if we remain committed to the process and focused on our goal, then we might be close to getting off that cold mountain to see the green valleys of Chile. I think this applies to all of us, so I'm going to write down 'Remain committed and focused.'"

"We had a bunch of players-only meetings at my high school," said Megan. "But none of them were like this."

"I can't say I've been in one like this either," Andrea concurred. "Normally, they're gripe sessions. Come to think of it, I probably did most of the complaining. But, so far, I've really liked the way this has been going."

There was a slight pause in the conversation, and so Tracy took the opportunity to share what was on her mind.

"Jasmine already mentioned how Piper is such an encourager, but I want to say something else about her that I think can apply to all of us. Well, I was talking with Piper in the training room yesterday after she hurt her knee. We all know she's a ball of energy and one of the hardest workers we've ever seen, but I realized those qualities don't need to be limited to just her. We can have all of us doing the same thing. It doesn't matter our talent level or status. I've decided that I'm going to try to be like Piper. I want to put forth as much effort as possible. I want to supply this team with energy. Because I spend so much time in the dugout during games, I'm going to call it 'Dugergy.'"

"That's awesome. I love it," said Haley. "I think you're right. It stinks that Piper is going to be out of commission, but we can all pick up the slack. We can all do this."

Haley then wrote the phrase 'Supply effort and energy' on the board.

Andrea then spoke up again. "Haley, I know I already mentioned my attitude in the traffic jam, but I wanted to mention something else I learned last night. For those who don't know, I was served a dessert called 'Humble Pie' yesterday when we stopped to eat. I thought I was right, but I was dead wrong. I saw a great example of servant leadership from the restaurant manager. It wasn't normal, or at least my normal. I realized how selfish I can be and how I can get obsessed with seeing just my tree and not the whole forest. I can get consumed with only my stuff. We need to serve each other. This concept will not be easy for me, but I realize I need to try and do better in this area."

Haley smiled big as she listened to Andrea speak. She remembered the scene from last night's restaurant.

"I was watching that whole thing from the other table and thought it was funny," said Haley. "Especially Zoe getting all red in the face and sweating because she ate a spicy sub. Glad you weren't allergic or anything, Zoe."

"Me too," said Zoe. "I might be a Vegan from here on out."

"Andrea, thanks for sharing," said Haley. "That's going to be a tough one for many of us, but we probably all need to think of each other a little bit more. We need to think about what's best for each other. This could be a key lesson as we look to finish the year strong, so I will list it with the others we've written down."

'Help and serve others' was written then on the board.

Gretchen then posed a question to her teammates, "How many of us want to admit that we aren't receptive to coaching?"

"That's a tough question," said Ava.

"Yes, it is," replied Gretchen. "But I've seen people in this room, including me sometimes, roll their eyes when our coaches ask us to do something new or try something new."

"Guilty!" Kylee said with a hand raised.

"I'm just asking if it's happened to you." continued Gretchen. "I've often been chewed out by my high school and travel coaches for not doing what they've been teaching. I've probably deserved it every time, even though I probably acted like I didn't deserve it. I'm sure every single time this happened, I passed the buck or didn't take responsibility for my own development as a player, like the first thing you wrote down."

"Hey, lose those excuses!" joked her roommate Libby.

"I know. That's what I'm saying," continued Gretchen. "I'm sure I made excuses, and they were probably good ones at the time, so what you guys listed as the first principle is very relevant to me. But when Brooklyn told that story about 'Mudita' and being happy when one of my teammates did something amazing, I realized that I've never responded that way. When I flip it around and think about all those times I've made mistakes, I blame it on someone else, like the pitcher, the coaches, or the umpire. I've had coaches tell me I'm uncoachable, and I normally blow it off or get defensive. I don't want to be that way. I understand, support, and encourage Mudita and can't wait to get the sticker on my helmet, but it's handling the mistakes I need help with. If you guys have any suggestions, please let me know, but I just thought I would mention it."

Haley asked Gretchen, "Would it be okay if I wrote it on the board? I think that's an important principle that can apply to all of us."

"Sure. It seems good. However, you want to sum up what I just said is fine with me," said Gretchen.

"Thanks for sharing. I'm going to put 'Improve and be coachable' because none of us know everything, and we can always get better, and the way most of us can get better is to be coachable."

"Sounds good to me," said Gretchen.

Haley looked at her watch, put down the marker, and then turned to her teammates.

"We've been here long enough, and I appreciate all the honesty and things you guys have said. This certainly has been one of the most productive meetings I've been a part of. I really wasn't prepared for this. Like I said, Kylee and I just wanted to share our thoughts on excuses and taking responsibility for our actions. I wasn't ready for all of you to share like you did, but it was awesome."

"Hey, Haley," said Ava. "I'm sorry to interrupt you, but you mentioned that you weren't prepared for what was going to be said at this meeting. That must have been a sign that you used that word. I wasn't going to say anything, but you said that word, and I think it's important."

"I agree, but why do you say it's important? What are you thinking?" Haley asked.

"The word *prepared* stood out to me because I wasn't prepared for the game yesterday. In fact, I'm rarely prepared because I don't play much. Zoe and I were talking, and she kind of lit into me about how my being unprepared can actually lead to me losing out on opportunities. It can also hurt the team, and you guys are my friends. Champions are prepared. Winners are prepared. I know some of us have not been taking things as seriously as we can. We haven't prepared as well as we can. I'm certainly at the top of that list, but I don't think it's a coincidence that we're playing badly and having a poor season. Whether it's practice, academics, sleep, conditioning, or anything else, we need to do better if we want to win."

I'm a freshman. I'm not the best player on this team. But this is a chance for me to be a voice and a leader on this team, Zoe thought.

"Ava is right," piped Zoe. "We have big games coming up, and our preparation might be the difference between winning and losing. I think Ava can be valuable to us moving forward if she is prepared. In fact, we can all be valuable to each other by being more prepared."

"My grandma has this little magnet thing on her refrigerator," Haley said. "It's some old guy from medieval times or something. His name is Sun Tzu, but he said, *The battle is won or lost before it is fought.* If we prepare a little harder and smarter, we might play above our talent level and win more. That was a good one. So, thanks, Ava."

'Prepare to win' became the tenth principle Haley wrote on the whiteboard. It was hard to believe that a team could learn so many crucial lessons in one day on one bus trip.

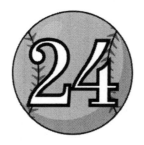

LEADERSHIP

The meeting was over, and a lot of great things were discussed. The team was feeling good about themselves when Zoe spoke up.

"Um, has anyone else noticed something about what we wrote down?"

Every set of eyeballs looked at the whiteboard and the ten principles that they listed, trying to figure out what Zoe had noticed.

It seemed like forever, but after a minute, Piper spoke up.

"I loved puzzles, and I'm seeing that whiteboard like one of those word puzzles I used to do on the back of those menus they'd have at restaurants for us kids. I see the word LEADERSHIP on that board."

"I see it now, too," Tracy said. "Wow, that's freaky. Is that what you saw, Zoe?"

"Sure is. That's some freaky stuff but also cool," said Zoe. "How's that for coincidences? It's almost like we were supposed to learn those lessons and write them down. Wow, how weird is that?"

Even though Zoe was the first to see the hidden word on the whiteboard, now every set of eyes saw it as clear as day. It was like they had just solved a hidden message with their super-secret decoder ring.

Lose the excuses

Excel in your role

Always be on time

Display a good attitude

Encourage team members

Remain committed & focused

Supply effort & energy

Help & serve others

Improve & be coachable

Prepare to win

"Regardless of how weird it is, that's a good lesson for us," said Megan. "Each of these things can apply to all of us. None of us are immune to any of those things. They all apply at some point. Also, each of us can do each one of those things. It's not like Haley is the only one who can improve and be coachable or that Gretchen is expected to be the only one who has to lose the excuses. Regardless of our status on the team, we can all can do these things."

"That's right. We can all be leaders," added Piper. "If we do those things, then we're demonstrating positive leadership. It will help the entire team. It's like leadership is the glue for all of these principles. Even though Haley and Kylee are our senior captains, we can all do these things. We can all practice and demonstrate leadership by doing these ten things."

"Since this is obviously like a big neon sign flashing at us saying be better and do better, what is our next step? How do we do these things now?" asked Zoe.

"First, we definitely need to take a picture of this," said Haley.

"Already did," Piper quickly replied.

"In that case, maybe we make a poster or something like that," suggested Kylee.

"I think that's a great idea. But let's do more," said Megan. "We already have some cool posters in our locker room. But we haven't been living up to those. I don't want this to end up the same."

"I don't think it would end up being ignored, so to speak because we actually came up with this stuff, not Coach," suggested Haley. "Don't get me wrong. His posters are pretty cool and say great things, but at the end of the day, they're his. However we did this, we actually came up with these things on our own. We can take ownership of the acronym thing. Sure, it should be a poster, but we need to be reminded of this often and live it out daily somehow."

"I agree. Last night's revelations and the things we came up with are too special to dismiss. This needs to be special somehow," said Piper.

"You mean like a blood oath?" joked Libby.

"We don't need to light candles or get out the knives," responded Haley. "Nothing creepy like that."

"How about we all sign the board like a contract, an agreement," suggested Zoe.

Kylee wasted no time, picked up two dry-erase markers, and tossed them to Libby and Gretchen.

"You guys were the first ones here today. Go ahead and be the first to sign the board."

Libby and Gretchen must have liked Zoe's idea because they didn't hesitate to get up from their seats and sign the board.

Each of the remaining players then took their turn signing the board in an unofficial covenant, setting their standards for the remainder of the season.

Piper announced to her teammates, "I just took another picture of the board. I wanted to get one with all of the signatures on it."

"Good idea," said Haley. "Send that to me, and I'll ask Coach to make it into a poster that goes right next to the door as we leave the locker room. That way, we'll see it every time we leave."

As she finished talking, Haley couldn't help but smile as she saw Jasmine raise her hand again.

"I thought I said there's no need to raise your hand."

"Uh, yeah, sorry. Anyway, I was thinking that your poster idea was cool. But we should also get something we can all have. Like mini posters in our lockers, t-shirts, wristbands, or something like that."

"I agree. Those are great ideas," Kylee said. "I actually like the wristband idea the best. Maybe we get the word LEADERSHIP on them in our school colors."

"And Coach might even let us wear them in practice," added Zoe. "That way, we'd constantly be reminding ourselves and each other just like the Mudita stickers."

"Great ideas, guys," said Haley. "I'll ask him about the wristbands and the poster."

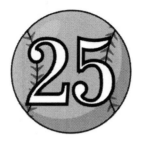

RIVALRY GAME

Practice the day before a game is normally more laid-back and involves a lot of fine-tuning. This was not a normal practice.

The players were more vocal than usual. Every rep in the batting cage was taken seriously. The tee work was crisp. Team situations were sharp. Players communicated between every pitch. Everyone was engaged. The energy was high. Sounds of 'Great throw,' 'Nice scoop,' 'Great pitch,' and 'Way to rip that ball' filled the practice field.

Piper, who had, in fact, torn her ACL, gave Coach a summary of yesterday's meeting. Coach Batdorff believed what was discussed was genuine, but he hadn't expected the principles to take hold this quickly.

"Great practice today! That's the way to bounce back from your last game."

Even though all the players were thinking about it, Kylee was the one who spoke first.

"We've dug ourselves quite a hole but are determined to finish the season strong. We know how we need to go about our business, Coach. We're sorry for how we've been handling ourselves this year, and that changes now."

"I appreciate that. I believe you ladies."

In all his years of coaching, Benny Batdorff had thought he'd seen it all. But the way this team approached today's practice was something unique. The way every member of the team, from freshman to senior, seemed to bring a different mentality. There might be something special to it.

"Make sure you ladies get some downtime tonight. Stay on top of your academics, but don't be late for dinner. We have a big game tomorrow."

"We got this, Coach!" the Eagles seemed to say in unison.

A little more than 24 hours later, the Eagles sat down next to their lockers after finishing up with their rivals, the Lakers. They weren't quite sure what Coach was going to say.

"The last time we met after a game, I was frustrated and wasn't hopeful about how the rest of this season would go. Tonight, I'm frustrated, but it's a different kind of frustration. I'm extremely hopeful."

Coach Batdorff took a sip of water and continued.

"I'm frustrated because you ladies battled tonight, and I wanted to see you get the 'W.' That probably would have been too much like a movie. But make no mistake. All those things you talked about were real. You might not have gotten rewarded on the scoreboard for the new attitude, but it was obvious to anyone watching that there was something different about you."

Coach Batdorff could tell they were glad he recognized them but still disappointed that they lost.

"You didn't win tonight on the scoreboard but won in my book. I know that might sound cheesy, but the truth is that you nearly beat an excellent Lakers team tonight. You had quality at-bats against one of the best pitchers in the league. You got their best hitter out three times. I also love how we dove for balls, sprinted out to our spots between innings, and no one took a called third strike. And Libby pitched her best game of the year. You ladies are trying to win the process of winning. You nearly pulled off the upset by doing the little things you hadn't been doing throughout the season. Imagine what can be done if we continue what we started the last couple of days. The good news is we have enough time left in the season to develop the kind of habits on the field that will match your attitudes."

Coach Batdorff picked up a dry-erase marker and approached the whiteboard, writing the word LEADERSHIP.

"This is what I saw tonight. I saw leadership. I saw teammates encouraging each other. I saw a high level of engagement and communication. I saw and heard amazing energy in the dugout. In the 7th inning, when it became clear we weren't going to pull the game out, I didn't detect any finger-pointing or blame being thrown around. I saw leadership from everyone, not just a senior, a starter, or a coach. As I said, I'm hopeful because I'm seeing genuine leadership from you."

Coach Batdorff paused and looked at the whiteboard. He pointed at the word LEADERSHIP and then at each of his players, saying their names aloud.

"Each of you can be a positive leader for us moving forward. This can still be a special season because, as you've already discovered, you're interconnected and responsible to one another on this journey. And make no mistake, it's a journey, not just a destination. You didn't win tonight but took a giant step forward on this journey together. I'm very, very proud of you. Now, bring it in."

The players got up from their seats quickly and met in the center of the locker room.

With an enthusiasm unmatched at any point in the season, the team said together, "1, 2, 3, TEAM."

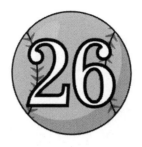

TOURNAMENT

The change in mentality and new habits were developed as the Eagles finished the regular season on a nine-game winning streak. Furthermore, that collection of players went deeper in the playoffs than any previous Eagles team had in school history.

After the final out had been made, ending their fantastic playoff run, the players walked into the locker room. Coach Batdorff addressed this group one last time and then let the seniors say a few words.

Doing her best to hold back her emotions, Haley spoke first.

"Okay, so we didn't win any championships during my four years. But I can obviously say that what we accomplished this year after starting as we did may have been more satisfying than winning any trophy. I will never forget the way we came together during this journey."

She couldn't believe the season and her softball career were over. But she felt at peace knowing that she had done what she could for the program.

"I'm so proud of you ladies," Haley went on. "I never wanted a season to continue more than I wanted this season to continue. Not because of the whole 'survive and advance' thing we all want at tournament time but because you're my family. We grew together this year, and that is something I'll never forget. Thanks, everyone!"

Then Kylee stood up and walked to the whiteboard on the wall.

"Until we had that team meeting, I never liked these things," she said, pointing at the whiteboard. "These boards were just something Coach would scribble on and write about things I didn't care about. That bus trip. That meeting the next day. That stuff changed my life. I know you don't expect me to be this deep, but it was about more than softball for me."

Kylee took off her wristband and repeatedly stretched it out in front of her teammates.

"This little thing reminds me every day that those ten things we learned on that bus trip and in that meeting are things that we can do no matter how much talent we have as a softball player, or in life, for that matter. I can apply all of those things to being a student, an employee one day, a wife or a mother."

Libby interrupted Kylee, "Wait, is there something you haven't told us?"

"Come on! I was pouring my heart out to you, and you have to go and make a joke."

"You're right. I'm sorry!"

Rolling her eyes and shaking her head, Kylee continued.

"Anyway, I'm a better person, not just a softball player, because I realized that I can display leadership in all aspects of my life. I can do those ten things in all areas of my life. Thanks for helping me see that."

Coach Batdorff walked over to her as Kylee approached her seat and hugged her.

"I'm so proud of you. I never thought I'd be saying this to you, but you were key to us making this tournament run. We're going to really miss you next year."

"Coach, you're going to make me cry. Stop that," said Kylee.

Coach Batdorff released his grip on Kylee but wasn't quite finished with her praise.

"Your stats might not win you a place in the record books, but we'll talk about your legacy for quite a while. Thanks for stepping up and taking responsibility."

From the corner of the locker room, Piper nudged forward on her crutches. "I know that I'm not a senior, but I wanted to say something quickly."

As one of the most respected people on the team and the entire campus, all eyes were now on Piper.

"I think I speak for the entire team when I say to the captains, thank you for showing us a great example of leadership and helping inspire us all to be good followers and to step up and be leaders ourselves."

Haley and Kylee nodded. They were appreciative of Piper and her words. She was already a positive leader; next year, she'd make a good team captain.

"As for you, Coach, thanks for trusting us enough and empowering us to develop as leaders. We learned that we're all on this journey together."

Piper adjusted her weight on the crutches before continuing.

"I wish this season weren't over, but the good news is our journey is still going on. I can't wait to have some recruits on campus, see our culture, and share the main thing we're about with them."

Coach Batdorff looked at Piper, picked up a marker, and then wrote something on the whiteboard.

"That's exactly right, Coach. That's the word. That's what we're all about. LEADERSHIP."

EAGLES

SUCCESS IS A CHOICE.
WE ALL CHOOSE TO BE BETTER!

1.) Lose the excuses
2.) Excel in your role
3.) Always be on time
4.) Display a good attitude
5.) Encourage team members
6.) Remain committed and focused
7.) Supply effort and energy
8.) Help and serve others
9.) Improve and be coachable
10.) Prepare to win

Libby _Piper_
Gretchen
Kylee
Brooklyn
Zoe
Ava
Tracy _HALEY_
Megan
Andrea
Jasmine

LEADERSHIP!

That's what
we're ALL about!

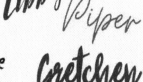

About Michael K. Thompson ...

Michael K. Thompson grew up in Charlevoix, Michigan. As an athlete, he participated in many sports, including football, baseball, and basketball, and has run more than a dozen marathons.

Michael earned a degree in English from Central Michigan University and is a Lambda Chi Alpha fraternity member. He always knew he wanted to stay close to athletics by being a coach.

Michael's coaching journey began after college when he discovered his passion for coaching fastpitch softball while teaching at Jonesville High School in Michigan. Over the past 25 years, he has honed his skills as a football and softball coach, currently teaching English and coaching softball at Frankfort High School in Frankfort, Michigan. His dedication and expertise were recognized when he was inducted into the Michigan High School Softball Coaches Hall of Fame in 2016.

As the owner of Great Lakes Sports Leadership, Michael works with coaches and student-athletes to develop leadership skills, accountability, character development, responsibility, team building, and to create championship team cultures. He hosts the "Leadership Matters" podcast about developing effective leadership skills and building a championship culture.

Michael is a licensed sports leadership facilitator through the Janssen Sports Leadership Center.

In his free time, Michael enjoys treasure hunting and coin collecting, showing his passion for discovery and history.

WEBSITE: GreatLakesSportsLeadership.com

TWITTER: @CoachMKThompson and @GLSLeadership

FACEBOOK: @GreatLakesSportsLeadership

INSTAGRAM: @GreatLakesSportsLeadership

Great Lakes Sports Leadership

Leadership, Culture, and Character

EMPOWERING THE NEXT
GENERATION

INTERESTED IN MICHAEL K.
THOMPSON SPEAKING AT YOUR
EVENT, WORKING WITH YOUR TEAM,
OR CONDUCTING A SUMMIT OR
WORKSHOP FOR YOUR
ORGANIZATION?

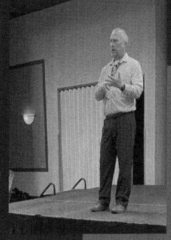

MICHAEL K. THOMPSON

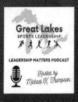

CHECK OUT THE "LEADERSHIP
MATTERS" PODCAST

 @CoachMKThompson
@GLSLeadership

 GreatLakesSportsLeadership

 Great Lakes Sports Leadership

GreatLakesSportsLeadership@gmail.com

GreatLakesSportsLeadership.com

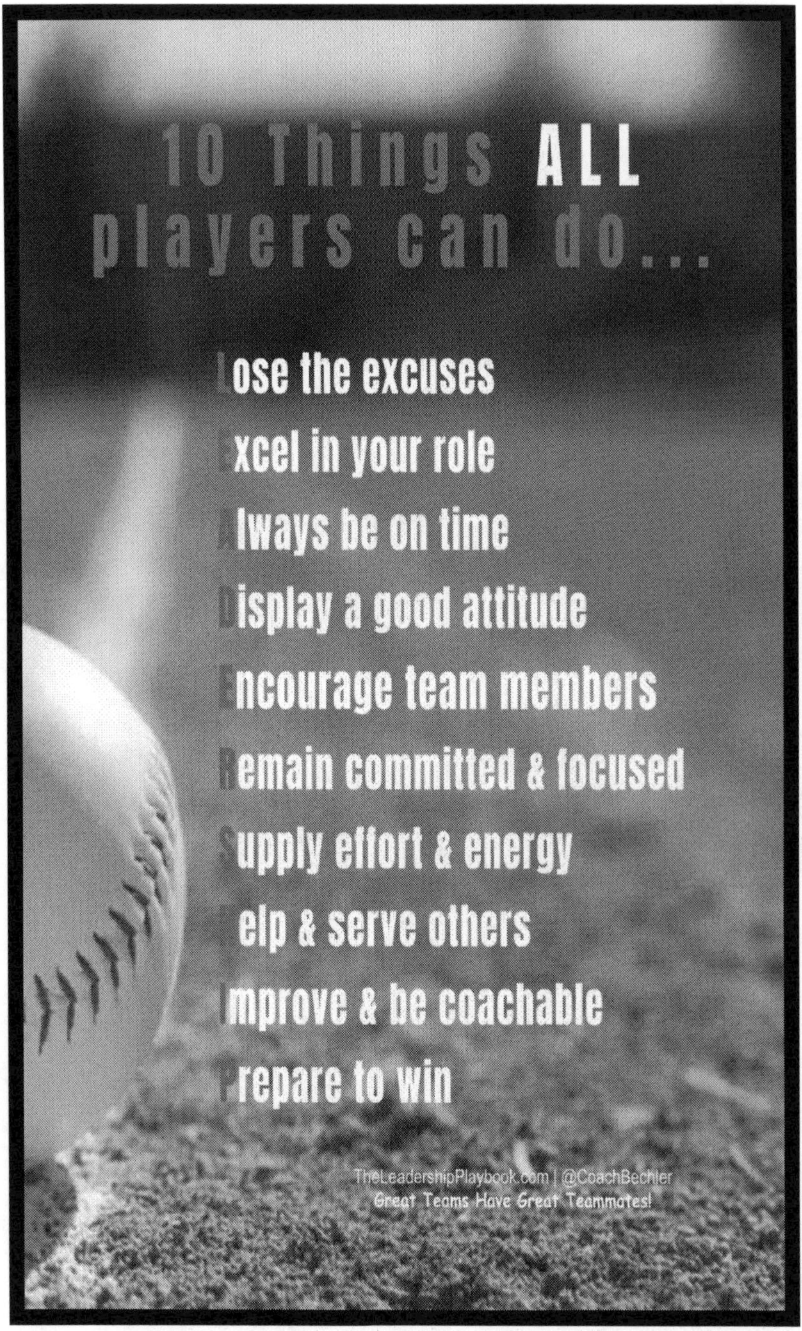

10 Things ALL players can do...

Lose the excuses

Excel in your role

Always be on time

Display a good attitude

Encourage team members

Remain committed & focused

Supply effort & energy

Help & serve others

Improve & be coachable

Prepare to win

TheLeadershipPlaybook.com | @CoachBechler
Great Teams Have Great Teammates!

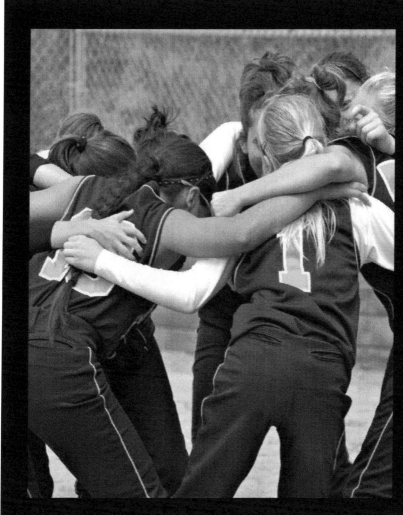

LEADERSHIP
that's what we're ALL about

TheLeadershipPlaybook.com
JAMY BECHLER

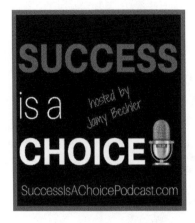
Merchandise Inspired by the Story

www.JamyBechler.com/Resources

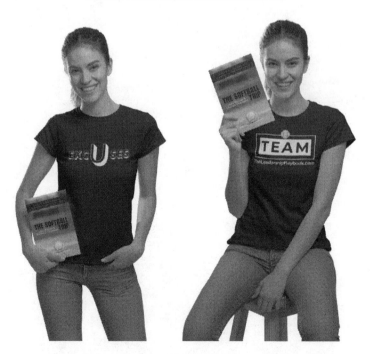

About Jamy Bechler ....

Jamy Bechler is a professional speaker, leadership consultant, author, and podcast host. He works with teams ranging from major corporations to the NBA. Before going into full-time leadership work, Jamy served for 20 years as a college basketball coach, professor, and administrator. When he hung up the whistle, he didn't stop coaching. He currently works with high-level organizations, teams, athletes, and coaches to help them maximize their potential in the area of leadership, culture, and teamwork.

Through his experiences as an athletic director, college coach, and leadership consultant, he has created TheLeadershipPlaybook.com, which is a membership site helping athletic departments develop better teammates, more positive leaders, and stronger cultures.

Jamy left his last college as the winningest coach in program history. His 2014 team earned the national "Champions of Character" award. He then moved to the high school ranks to serve as an athletic director for two years. As an athletic director, he transformed the athletic department, instituting budgeting processes, student-athlete leadership training, and innovative marketing strategies that were featured in Athletic Management magazine. He supervised the 5th largest high school gymnasium in the country and oversaw the boys basketball team winning their 8th state championship (most in Indiana history).

Jamy is the host of the "Success is a Choice" podcast, which highlights individuals from various industries and walks of life. Guests have included Clark Kellogg, Rachel Cruze, Dwane Casey, Kara Lawson, Kevin Harrington, Mike Lombardi, Sue Enquist, Bill Curry, and Phil Hellmuth to name just a few. The John Maxwell certified leadership coach also appears as a guest expert on various podcasts ranging from sports, leadership, politics, education, and business.

In addition to being a high school athletic director, Jamy has coached or played at the NCAA-I, II, III, and NAIA levels. As a student-athlete at Hiram College, he earned varsity letters in three different sports (football, basketball, and track) at various points in his collegiate career.

Jamy and his wife, Tabitha, have one son, Jaylen, whom they adopted at birth. They live near Akron, Ohio. He also belongs to a number of civic and community organizations including the NAACP, the Fellowship of Christian Athletes, the Pro Football Hall of Fame Booster Club, Barberton Community Turf Committee, National Sales & Marketing Executives, YMCA, Akron Chamber of Commerce, Kiwanis and Rotary.

Resources from Jamy Bechler

www.JamyBechler.com/Resources

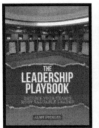
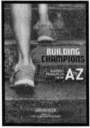
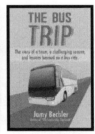
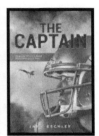

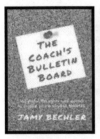
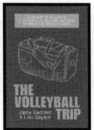
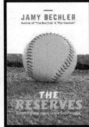
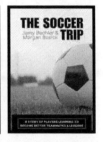

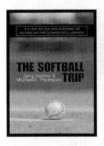
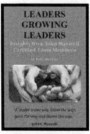
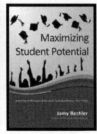
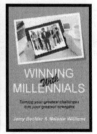

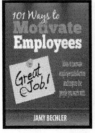
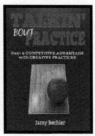
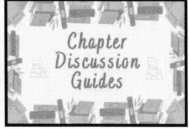

SUCCESS IS A CHOICE
WHAT CHOICE WILL YOU MAKE TODAY?

Interested in Jamy Bechler speaking at your event, working with your team, or conducting a workshop for your organization?

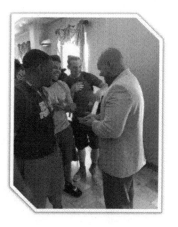

LinkedIn: JamyBechler

Twitter: @CoachBechler

Instagram: @CoachBechler

Facebook: JamyBechlerLeadership

Email speaking@JamyBechler.com

Visit TheLeadershipPlaybook.com and join the 1000's of athletes & coaches improving their leadership skills.

Use coupon code "Trip" to receive a 25% discount on your membership.

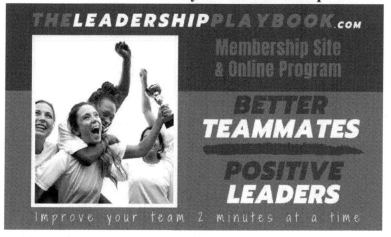

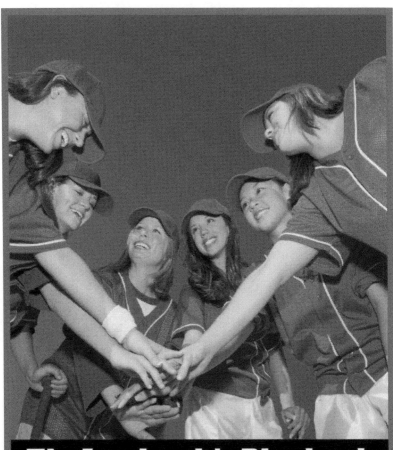

TheLeadershipPlaybook.com

Positive LEADERS
Better TEAMMATES
Stronger CULTURES

GREAT TEAMS HAVE GREAT TEAMMATES!

Made in the USA
Columbia, SC
26 November 2024

47412557R00078